Copyright © 2021 by Gary McMorrow -All rights reserved.

No part of this publication may be reproduced, distributed, or transmitted in any form or by any means, including photocopying, recording, or other electronic or mechanical methods, without the prior written permission of the publisher, except in the case of brief quotations embodied in reviews and certain other non-commercial uses permitted by copyright law.

This Book is provided with the sole purpose of providing relevant information on a specific topic for which every reasonable effort has been made to ensure that it is both accurate and reasonable. Nevertheless, by purchasing this Book you consent to the fact that the author, as well as the publisher, are in no way experts on the topics contained herein, regardless of any claims as such that may be made within. It is recommended that you always consult a professional prior to undertaking any of the advice or techniques discussed within.This is a legally binding declaration that is considered both valid and fair by both the Committee of Publishers Association and the American Bar Association and should be considered as legally binding within the United States.

CONTENTS

BRUNCH & SIDE DISHES RECIPES 7
- Cheesy Omelet Cups 7
- Eggs En Cocotte 7
- Cream Of Potato Soup 7
- Eggs & Red Beans Casserole 7
- Golden Beets With Green Olives 7
- Steamed Scotch Eggs 7
- Classic Mushroom Stroganoff 8
- Traditional Provençal Ratatouille 8
- Quinoa Mushroom Salad 8
- Mushroom Pâté 8
- Electric Pressure Cooker Huevos Rancheros ... 9
- Orange Marmalade Oatmeal 9
- Scrambled Eggs With Cranberries & Mint ... 9
- Broccoli With Italian-style Mayonnaise 9
- Chicken Sandwiches With Bbq Sauce 9
- Grapefruit Potatoes With Walnuts 10
- Vegetable Frittata With Cheddar & Ricotta ... 10
- Warm Spinach Salad With Eggs & Nuts 10
- Tasty Onion Frittata With Bell Pepper 10
- Vegan Baked Beans 10
- Tasty Asparagus Soup 10
- Eggplant With Steamed Eggs And Tomatoes .. 11
- French Balsamic Peppers 11
- Light & Fruity Yogurt 11
- Chili Deviled Eggs 11
- Steamed Artichoke 11
- Morning Frittatas 12
- Garlic Eggs 12
- Squash Tart Oatmeal 12
- Eggs Mushroom Casserole 12
- Vegetables With Halloumi Cheese 12
- Egg Caprese Breakfast 13
- Lazy Steel Cut Oats With Coconut Milk 13
- Braised Collard Greens With Bacon 13
- Mediterranean Tomato Soup With Feta Cheese 13
- Brussel Sprouts With Onions & Apples 13
- Italian Stuffed Peppers With Mushroom And Sausage 14
- Bacon And Cheese Crustless Quiche 14
- Green Soup With Navy & Pinto Beans 14
- Effortless Tomato-lentil Soup 14
- Spinach Hash 14
- Chicken & Vegetable Rice Soup 15
- Coco Quinoa Bowl 15
- Garam Masala Parsnip & Red Onion Soup ... 15
- Perfect Mediterranean Asparagus 15
- Asian Vegetable Soup 15
- Lentil-arugula Pancake 16
- Winter Vegetable And Lentil Stew 16
- Frittata With Vegetables & Cheese 16
- Goat Cheese & Beef Egg Scramble 16
- Delicious Chicken & Potato Soup 17
- Mushroom-spinach Cream Soup 17
- Cheddar Baked Eggs 17
- Gourmet Cilantro Salmon 17
- French Baked Eggs 17
- Garden Vegetable Soup 17
- Green Beans Salad 18
- Electric Pressure Cooker Bread Pudding 18
- Avocado Quinoa Salad 18
- Black Bean And Egg Casserole 18
- Meat-free Lasagna With Mushrooms 18
- Easy Homemade Omelet 19
- Chickpea Hummus 19
- Moroccan-style Couscous Salad 19
- Coconut Porridge 19
- Maple-orange Glazed Root Vegetables 19
- Honey-mustard Glazed Cipollini Onions ... 20
- Fresh Red Beets 20
- Spanish Omelet 20
- Lentil And Carrot Soup 20
- Lime Potatoes 20
- Quick Mushroom-quinoa Soup 20
- Instant Sweet Potato 21
- Strawberry Compote 21
- Rustic Soup With Turkey Balls & Carrots ... 21
- Garam Masala Eggs 21
- Cheesy Grits With Crispy Pancetta 21
- Glazed Baby Carrots 21
- Goat Cheese & Beef Steak Salad 22
- Breakfast Cobbler 22

SOUPS, STEWS & CHILIS RECIPES 23
- Chicken And Kale Soup 23
- Piri Piri Chicken Soup 23
- Simple Clam Chowder 23
- Spiced Sweet Potato Soup 23
- Jalapeño Chicken Soup With Tortilla Chips ... 23
- Fall Bean Chili 24
- Bengali Parsnip Soup 24
- Quick Chicken Soup 24
- Root Vegetable Stew 24
- Pumpkin & Pearl Barley Soup 24
- Spicy Broccoli And Cheese Soup 25
- Chicken Noodle Soup 25
- Cheesy Tomato Soup 25
- Gingered Squash Soup 25
- Simple Chicken And Kale Soup 25
- Rich And Easy Chicken Purloo 26
- Parsley Pork Chili 26
- Cashew & Tomato Soup 26
- "eat-me" Ham And Pea Soup 26
- Cheesy Cauliflower Soup 26
- Thai Coconut Curry Stew 26
- Grandma's Noodle Soup 27
- Chickpea & Spinach Chili 27
- Authentic Kentucky Burgoo 27
- Veal And Buckwheat Groat Stew 27
- Pecorino Mushroom Soup 28
- Black Bean Soup 28
- Gingery Butternut Squash Soup 28
- Turkey & Vegetable Stew 28
- Authentic French Onion Soup 28

Recipe	Page
Chicken Spinach Corn Soup	28
Tofu And Miso Soup	29
Rice And Beef Soup	29
Ethiopian Spinach And Lentil Soup	29
Ham And Potato Soup	29
Vegan Pottage Stew	30
Autumn Pumpkin Soup	30
Creamy Mushroom Soup With Chicken	30
Green Bean Soup	30
Fast Chicken Rice Soup	30
Bean And Ham Soup	31
Two-cheese Carrot Sauce	31
Borscht Beet Soup	31
Peppery Ground Pork Soup	31
Old-fashioned Duck Soup With Millet	31
Thai Tom Saap Pork Ribs Soup	31
Bacon And Veggie Soup	32
Hearty Beef Soup	32
Mushroom Chicken Soup	32
Kale And Veal Stew	32
Easy Veggie Soup	32
Seafood And Vegetable Ragout	33
Kale, Potato & Beef Stew	33
Electric Pressure Cooker Ham And Potato Soup	33
Mom's Pork Vegetable Soup	33
Coconut Seafood Soup	33
Chicken, Shrimp And Sausage Gumbo	34
Chicken Soup With Vegetables	34
Seafood Chowder With Bacon And Celery	34
Hearty Irish Burgoo	35
Beef Borscht Soup	35
Three Beans Mix Chili	35
Butternut Squash Curry Soup	35
Japanese-style Tofu Soup	35
Veggie Cheese Soup	36
Cheddar Cheese And Broccoli Soup	36
Vegetable Mediterranean Delight Stew	36
Easy Vegetarian Ratatouille	36
Chicken & Noodle Soup	36
Potato And Corn Soup	37
Chinese-style Chicken Stew With Broccoli	37
Beef And Cabbage Soup	37
Butternut Squash & Apple Soup	37
Meatball Soup	38
Vegetarian Minestrone With Navy Beans	38
Lentil & Bell Pepper Soup	38
Corn And Potato Chowder	38
Minestrone Soup	38
Leek Soup With Tofu	39
VEGETABLE & VEGETARIAN RECIPES	**40**
Onion & Chickpea Stew	40
Steamed Vegetables	40
Cheesy Potatoes With Herbs	40
Easy Vegan Posole	40
Sautéed Spinach & Leeks With Blue Cheese	40
Vegetable One-pot	40
Zucchini And Bell Pepper Stir Fry	41
Spicy Pickled Potatoes	41
Mixed Vegetables Medley	41
Electric Pressure Cooker French Onion Soup	41
Maple-glazed Acorn Squash	41
Pumpkin & Potato Mash	42
Tomato, Lentil & Quinoa Stew	42
Flavorful Vegetable Mix	42
Indian Coconut Kale Curry	42
Sumac Red Potatoes	42
Indian Dhal With Veggies	42
Elegant Farro With Greens & Pine Nuts	42
Pumpkin Puree	43
Buttery Mashed Cauliflower	43
Egg & Ham Traybake	43
Savory Spinach And Leek Relish	43
Spicy Vegetable Salsa	43
Parsnips & Cauliflower Mash	43
Feta & Nut Green Beans	44
Meat Lover's Omelet	44
Beets And Cheese	44
Indian Lentils Dhal	44
Cauliflower Salad With Mozzarella Cheese	44
Mom's Carrots With Walnuts & Berries	45
Poblano Pepper & Sweet Corn Side Dish	45
Broccoli Leeks Green Soup	45
Asparagus And Mushrooms	45
Quick Indian Creamy Eggplant	45
Steamed Artichokes & Green Beans With Mayo Dip	45
Creamy Spinach Tagliatelle With Mushrooms	46
Easy Homemade Pizza	46
Creamy Artichoke, Garlic, And Zucchini	46
Steamed Artichokes With Mayo Dip	46
Lime & Ginger Eggplants	46
Palak Paneer	47
Tomato & Apple Cider Infused Ratatouille	47
Power Green Minestrone Stew With Lemon	47
Easy Vegan Pizza	47
Vegetarian Chipotle Stew	47
Arabic-style Cauliflower Salad	48
Delicious Mushroom Goulash	48
Lentil & Carrot Chili	48
Electric Pressure Cooker Cauliflower Curry	48
Carrot Vegan Gazpacho	48
Electric Pressure Cooker Steamed Artichoke	48
English Vegetable Potage	49
Veggie Flax Patties	49
Steamed Artichoke With Garlic Mayo Sauce	49
Steamed Vegetables Side Dish	49
Carrot & Chickpea Boil With Cherry Tomatoes	49
Sage Cauliflower Mash	49
Parmesan Lentil Spread	50
Parmesan & Veggie Mash	50
Potato Spinach Corn Mix	50
Electric Pressure Cooker Basic Steamed Vegetables	50
Cabbage With Carrot	50
Pure Basmati Rice Meal	51
Cauliflower & Potato Curry With Cilantro	51
Mirin Tofu Bowl	51
Steamed Paprika Broccoli	51

Celery & Red Bean Stew	51
Spinach & Mushroom Tagliatelle	51
Broccoli, Cauliflower & Zucchini Cakes	52
Puréed Chili Carrots	52
Vegetable Medley With Brazil Nuts	52
Sweet Potato Medallions With Garlic & Rosemary	52
Spanish-style "tortilla De Patatas"	52
Crushed Potatoes With Aioli	53
Vegetarian Khoreshe Karafs (persian Celery Stew)	53
Kale And Sweet Potatoes With Tofu	53
Garlic & Leek Cannellini Beans	53
Maple Glazed Carrots	53
Hearty French Ratatouille	53
Monday Night Rice With Red Beans	54

BEEF & LAMB, PORK RECIPES 55

Burrito Beef	55
Tagliatelle With Beef Sausage & Beans	55
Green Chili Pork With Pomodoro Sauce	55
Zucchini & Potato Beef Stew	55
Thyme Creamy Beef Roast	55
Jalapeño Ground Pork Stew	56
European Stew	56
Savory Baby Back Ribs	56
Savory Beef Roast In Passion Fruit Gravy	56
Spinach, Rice And Beef Sausage Stew	56
Greek-style Cooked Pulled Pork	57
Sage Pork Butt With Potatoes	57
Ground Pork Soup With Leeks & Carrots	57
Butternut Squash Beef With Bok Choy	57
Awesome Rutabaga And Pear Pork Loins	57
Mediterranean Tomato Beef Soup	57
Mount-watering Beef Ribs With Shiitake	58
Lamb Shanks In Port Wine	58
Dinner Ribs With Beets And Potatoes	58
Pork Shoulder Roast With Noodles	58
Sliced Beef Steak With Carrots	58
Sweet Shredded Pork	59
Mom's Rump Roast With Potatoes	59
Chili Beef Brisket With Chives	59
Sage Pork Ribs In Pecan Sauce	59
Quick Pork Chops With Cabbage	59
Lamb With Green Onions	59
Tender Bbq Ribs	59
Pork Ribs With Tomato And Carrots	60
Pork Chops With Sage	60
Pork With Prune Sauce	60
Autumn Beef Stew	60
Spiced Beef Brisket & Pancetta Stew	60
Beef And Sauerkraut Dinner	61
Beef Paprikash	61
Pancetta & Cheese Rigatoni	61
Saucy Beef Short Ribs	61
Lamb Cacciatore	61
Tasty Beef With Carrot-onion Gravy	61
Sunday Beef Roast With Garam Masala	62
Curried Pork Stew With Peas	62
Veggie Beef Steak With Beer Sauce	62
Pork Shoulder In Bbq Sauce	62
Cilantro Vegetable Beef Soup	62
Picante Beef Stew With Barley	63
Lamb & Mushroom Ragout	63
Pork & Mushrooms	63
Cuban Style Pork	63
Sweet & Sour Pork	63
Herbed Veggie Beef Rib Eye	64
Pineapple & Soda-glazed Ham	64
Juicy Chorizo Sausage With Tater Tots	64
Cheese Beef Taco Pie	64
Pork Soup With Red Wine	64
Pork Infused With Orange Juice	64
Papaya Short Ribs	65
Pork Meatballs With Sour Mushroom Sauce	65
Hungarian Bean Soup	65
Beef Roast With Onions	65
Pork Chops With Broccoli	65
Well-made Cheesy Meatballs	66
Pork Chops With Veggies	66
Country Beef Stew With Sweet Potatoes	66
Chorizo With Bell Peppers & Onions	66
Pork Steaks With Apricot Sauce	66
Pear Pork Tenderloin	66
Pork Shoulder Infused With Lime & Mint	67
Fall Pork Loin Chops With Red Cabbage	67
Pork Chops In Cream Of Mushrooms	67
Pork Sandwiches	67
Thyme Braised Lamb Shanks	67
Beef & Tomato Curry	67
Winter Beef With Vegetables	68
Ribs With Plum Sauce	68
Juniper Beef Ragu	68
Asian-style Flank Steaks	68
Pork City Pot	68
Garlicky Bbq Pork Butt	69
Sausage With Beer & Sauerkraut	69
Mexican-style Ropa Vieja	69

POULTRY RECIPES 70

Chicken Fricassee	70
Fettuccine With Duck Ragout	70
Chicken Curry (ver. 1)	70
Allspice Turkey Drumsticks With Beer	70
Simple Chicken Thighs	70
Sweet Saucy Chicken	70
Bell Pepper & Carrot Chicken Stew	71
Cheesy Chicken Tenders	71
Bacon And Cheese Quiche	71
Chicken With Black Beans	71
Salsa Verde Chicken	71
Pilaf With Zucchini & Chicken	72
Orange & Red Pepper Infused Chicken	72
Drumsticks In Adobo Sauce	72
Turkey Stew With Root Vegetables	72
Creamy Chicken With Tomato Sauce	73
Homemade Turkey Burgers	73
Rich Meatball Soup	73
Lemony Chicken With Red Currants	73
Spring Onion Buffalo Wings	73
Tender Chicken With Garden Vegetables	74

- Savory Chicken Wings With Worcestershire Sauce 74
- Creamed Taco Chicken Salad 74
- Mom's Orange Chicken 74
- Chicken With Port Wine Sauce 75
- Chicken Drumsticks With Potatoes & Veggies 75
- Cannellini & Sausage Stew 75
- Cumin Shredded Chicken 75
- Hard-boiled Eggs 75
- Chicken Congee 76
- Chicken & Mushrooms With White Wine 76
- Tarragon Whole Chicken 76
- Easy Teriyaki Chicken 76
- Pumpkin & Wild Rice Cajun Chicken 76
- Juicy Turkey With Mushrooms 77
- Momma's Chicken With Salsa Verde 77
- Country Chicken With Vegetables 77
- Spicy Honey Chicken 77
- Traditional Locrio De Pollo 77
- Cranberry Turkey With Hazelnuts 78
- Fabulous Orange Chicken Stew 78
- Asian Garlic And Honey Chicken 78
- Chicken With Artichokes And Bacon 78
- Buttered Chicken With Artichokes & Rosemary 78
- Easy Millet And Chicken Bowl 79
- Easy Spicy Chicken Wings 79
- Cheesy Chicken Quinoa 79
- Electric Pressure Cooker Chicken Creole 79
- Saucy Chicken Teriyaki 80
- Turkey With Smoked Paprika 80
- Asian-style Chicken 80
- Peppered Chicken With Chunky Salsa 80
- Rosemary Whole Chicken With Asparagus Sauce 80
- Sage Chicken With Potatoes & Snow Beans 81
- Egg And Potato Mayo Salad 81
- Thanksgiving Turkey Breasts 81
- Classic Lemon Chicken 81
- Fried Turkey Meatballs With Pasta 81
- Smoky Paprika Chicken 82
- Awesome Chicken In Tikka Masala Sauce 82
- Sesame Chicken Teriyaki 82
- Chicken Siciliano With Marsala Wine 82
- Shredded Chicken With Marinara 83
- Sage Chicken In Orange Gravy 83
- Sticky Sesame Chicken 83
- Paprika Rosemary Chicken 83
- Whole Chicken With White Wine 83
- Green Chili Chicken 84
- Tasty Indian Chicken Curry 84
- Rice & Lentil Chicken With Parsley 84
- Chicken Marrakesh 84
- Chicken In Garlic-mustard Sauce 84
- Chicken Salsa 85
- Garlic Chicken 85
- Turkey With Garlic Herb Sauce 85
- Turkey Fillets With Cremini Mushrooms 85
- Chicken With Cheese Parsley Dip 85
- Quick Swiss Chard & Chicken Stew 86
- Creole Chicken With Rice 86
- Easy Italian Chicken Stew With Potatoes 86

FISH & SEAFOOD RECIPES 87
- Indian Meen Kulambu 87
- Old Bay Crab 87
- Chickpea & Olives Seafood Pot 87
- Herby Trout Fillets With Olives 87
- Salmon With Parsley-lemon Sauce 87
- Seafood With Halloumi Cheese And Olives 87
- Cá Kho Tộ (caramelized & Braised Fish) 88
- Coconut Cod Curry 88
- Cheesy Tuna 88
- Cod Meal 88
- Old Bay Fish Tacos 88
- Mahi-mahi With Tomatoes 89
- American Clam Chowder 89
- Salmon With Pecan Coating 89
- Fish Packs 89
- Steamed Mussels In Scallion Sauce 89
- Simple Steamed Salmon Fillets 90
- Brussels Sprout Shrimp 90
- Mediterranean Cod With Cherry Tomatoes 90
- Delicious Cod With Cherry Tomatoes 90
- Basil Salmon With Artichokes & Potatoes 90
- Electric Pressure Cooker Mediterranean Fish 91
- Shrimp And Beans Mix 91
- Extraordinary Greek-style Fish 91
- Halibut With Cheese-mayo Sauce 91
- Mediterranean Cod With Olives 92
- Haddock Fillets With Steamed Green Beans .. 92
- White Wine Oysters 92
- Mustardy Steamed Catfish Fillets 92
- Clam & Prawn Paella 92
- Tunisian-style Couscous 93
- Canned Tuna Casserole 93
- Steamed Halibut Packets 93
- Seafood Platter 93
- Vietnamese-style Caramel Fish 93
- Electric Pressure Cooker Lobster Roll 94
- Codfish And Tomato Casserole 94
- Spicy Haddock Curry 94
- Chili-lime Shrimps 94
- Orange-butter Sea Bass 94
- Spicy Thai Prawns 95
- Collard Greens Octopus & Shrimp 95
- Citrus Marinated Smelt With Okra & Cherry Tomatoes 95
- Buttery Mackerel With Peppers 95
- Louisiana-style Seafood Boil 95
- Egg Noodles & Cheese With Tuna & Peas 96
- Easy Mahi Mahi With Enchilada Sauce 96
- Beer-steamed Mussels 96
- Lemon & Herbs Stuffed Tench 96
- Tuna With Egg 96
- Mussels With Wine-scallion Sauce 96
- Flounder With Dill And Capers 97
- Salmon Zucchini Stew 97
- The Ultimate Crab Patties 97
- Vermouth Tilapia Medley 97
- Greek Kakavia Fish Soup 97

Lemon White Fish	98
Mix-and-match Fish Packets	98
Tuna With Lemon And Eschalot	98
Herbed Carp Risotto	98
Seafood Paella	98
Electric Pressure Cooker Boiled Octopus	99
Delicious Shrimp Salad	99
Shrimp Curry	99
Parsley Squid	99
Shrimp Scampi	99
Steamed Fish Patra Ni Maachi	99
Salmon With Green Peas & Rice	100
Steamed Trout With Garlic & Fresh Herbs	100
Alfredo Tuscan Shrimp	100
Sea Scallops In Champagne Sauce	100
Soy Sauce Cheese Shrimp Scampi	100
Sea Scallops With Champagne Butter Sauce	100
Seafood Traditional Spanish Paella	101
Tiger Prawns Paella	101
Sole With Tartar Sauce	101
Vegetable Salmon Skewers	101
Green Lemon Salmon	102
Spinach & Trout With Red Sauce	102

SNACKS & DESSERTS, APPETIZERS RECIPES 103

Basil Infused Avocado Dip	103
Berry Mix, Mango And Apple Sauce	103
Cinnamon-flavored Apple Sauce	103
Allspices Cake	103
Easy Peach Cobbler	103
Cheesy Breakfast Potatoes	103
Duck Legs With Serrano Pepper Sauce	103
Cauliflower Popcorn	104
Spinach Dip	104
Peanut Pear Wedges	104
Coconut & Orange Cheesecake	104
Beef Ribs Texas Bbq Style	104
Lemony Berry Cream	104
Simple Cranberry Chocolate Biscuits	105
Swiss Chard Crisps With Orange Juice	105
Herby Cipollini Onions	105
Pineapple Chocolate Pudding	105
Holiday Almond Cake	105
Thyme Tomato Sauce	105
Almond Butter Lemon Pears	106
Apple Coconut Dessert	106
Tasty Apple Risotto	106
Awesome Chocolate Lava Cake	106
Rose Rice Pudding With Nuts	106
Sausage & Cream Cheese Dip	106
Teriyaki Chicken In Lettuce Wrap	106
Yummy Smoked Sausages	107
Party Cinnamon & Yogurt Cheesecake	107
Christmas Banana Bread	107
Dijon Deviled Eggs	107
Best Bacon Wrapped Mini Smokies	107
Cheesy Hamburger Dip	107
Almond Butter Bars	108
Mayonnaise & Bacon Stuffed Eggs	108
Pineapple Upside Down Cake	108
Amazing White Chocolate Fondue	108
Cashew Cholocate Spread	108
Apricot, Pear And Cherry Compote	108
Apple Coffee Cake	109
Cheese Sweet Corn	109
Fall Root Vegetable Mix	109
Chocolate Pudding Cake	109
Smoked Paprika Potato Chips	109
Pumpkin Hummus	109
Quick Rum Egg Custard	110
Silky Lemon Cheesecake With Blueberries	110
Zesty Carrots With Pistachios	110
Mom's Banana Cake	110
Chocolate-strawberry Bars	110
Sticky Sweet Chicken Wings	111
Bacon Asparagus Wraps	111
Tasty Honey Pumpkin Pie	111
Scrumptious Stuffed Pears	111
White Chocolate Cake In A Cup	111
Grandma's Pear And Peach Compote	111
Pumpkin Custard	111
Authentic Spanish Crema Catalana	112
Cheese Fondue	112
Hot Chicken Dip	112
Zucchini Potato Patties	112
Coconut Stuffed Apples	112
Sticky Bbq Chicken Drumsticks	112
Cinnamon & Raisin Muffins	112
Apple Cacao Dessert	113
Cremini Mushrooms With Sesame Paste	113
Chicken Noodle Dip	113
Homemade Raspberry Compote	113
Simple Poached Apricots	113
Orange Dip	113
Crispy Potato Sticks	113
Ice Cream Topped Brownie Cake	114
Cannellini Bean & Chili Dip	114

APPENDIX : RECIPES INDEX 115

BRUNCH & SIDE DISHES RECIPES

Cheesy Omelet Cups

INGREDIENTS for Servings: 2

4 eggs	½ tsp Italian
½ cup cheddar cheese, crumbled	seasoning mix
½ small onion, finely chopped	Salt and black pepper, to serve
	2 tbsp heavy cream

DIRECTIONS and Cooking Time: 10 Minutes
In a bowl, mix eggs, salt, pepper, and heavy cream. Whisk until well combined and add the remaining ingredients. Add 1 cup of water and lay the steam rack. Lower the ramekins on the steam rack and seal the lid. Cook on High Pressure for 6 minutes. When ready, do a quick release. Serve hot.

Eggs En Cocotte

INGREDIENTS for Servings: 3

Butter or cooking spray	1 tablespoon chives
3 tablespoons cream	Salt and pepper to taste
3 eggs	

DIRECTIONS and Cooking Time: 20 Minutes
Place a steamer rack in the Electric Pressure Cooker and pour a cup of water. Grease three ramekins with butter or cooking spray. Place 1 tablespoon of cream in each ramekin. Carefully crack an egg into each ramekin.5. Sprinkle with chives and season with salt and pepper on top. Place on the steamer rack. Close the lid and press the Manual button. Adjust the cooking time to 20 minutes. Do natural pressure release.

Cream Of Potato Soup

INGREDIENTS for Servings: 4

1 pound potatoes, cut into bite-sized pieces	2 garlic cloves, minced
1 cup double cream	Kosher salt and ground black pepper, to taste
1 sweet pepper, deveined and sliced	1/2 teaspoon cayenne pepper
1 jalapeno pepper, deveined and sliced	4 tablespoons all-purpose flour
3 cups creamed corn kernels	4 cups vegetable broth
1 sweet onion, chopped	2 tablespoons butter

DIRECTIONS and Cooking Time: 25 Minutes
Press the "Sauté" button and melt the butter. Once hot, sauté the sweet onions, garlic, and peppers for about 3 minutes or until they are tender and fragrant. Sprinkle the flour over the vegetables; continue stirring approximately 4 minutes or until your vegetables are coated. Add the broth and potatoes and gently stir to combine. Secure the lid. Choose the "Manual" mode and cook for 5 minutes at High pressure. Once cooking is complete, use a quick pressure release; carefully remove the lid. Press the "Sauté" button and use the lowest setting. Stir in the creamed corn, double cream, salt, black pepper, and cayenne pepper. Let it simmer, stirring continuously for about 5 minutes or until everything is thoroughly heated. Taste and adjust the seasonings. Bon appétit!

Eggs & Red Beans Casserole

INGREDIENTS for Servings: 3

3 eggs	½ cup cheddar cheese shredded
1 cup water	½ cup red beans, boiled
½ small onion chopped	Sea salt and pepper, to taste
½ cup cooked ham or bacon	
¼ cup heavy cream	

DIRECTIONS and Cooking Time: 20 Minutes
Add 1 cup of water to the Electric Pressure Cooker and place the trivet inside. Add all the ingredients to a bowl except the cheese and whisk well. Take a heatproof container and pour the egg mixture into it. Place the container over the trivet.5. Secure the lid of the cooker and press the "Manual" function key. Adjust the time to 20 minutes and cook at high pressure. After the beep, release the pressure naturally and remove the lid. Drizzle the shredded cheese on top and serve hot.

Golden Beets With Green Olives

INGREDIENTS for Servings: 4

4 golden beets	1 tsp garlic, minced
1 tbsp olive oil	2 tbsp balsamic vinegar
10 green olives	Salt and black pepper to taste
1 tbsp chopped parsley	

DIRECTIONS and Cooking Time: 30 Minutes
Place beets in the pressure cooker and cover with water. Seal the lid and cook on Manual for 20 minutes at High. Release the pressure quickly. Let the beets cool. Whisk together the remaining ingredients in a bowl. Slice beets and combine with dressing, to serve.

Steamed Scotch Eggs

INGREDIENTS for Servings: 4

| 4 large eggs | 1 tablespoon vegetable oil |
| 1-pound ground beef | |

DIRECTIONS and Cooking Time: 12 Minutes

Place a steamer basket in the Electric Pressure Cooker and add a cup of water. Place the eggs in the steamer basket and close the lid. Press the Steam button and adjust the cooking time to 6 minutes. Once the timer beeps, do natural pressure release and take the eggs out. Place the eggs in an ice bath to arrest the cooking process. When the eggs are cool, remove the shells. Set aside. Divide the ground beef into four and flatten using your hands. Place the boiled egg in the middle and cover the entire egg with the ground beef. Do the same thing on the rest of the eggs. Set aside. Press the Sauté button on the Electric Pressure Cooker and add the oil. Once the oil is hot, brown the Scotch eggs on four sides. Set aside.7. Place a steam rack in the Electric Pressure Cooker and pour in a cup of water. Place the browned scotch eggs on the steamer rack and close the lid. Press the Manual button and adjust the cooking time to 6 minutes. Do natural pressure release.

Classic Mushroom Stroganoff

INGREDIENTS for Servings: 8

14 ounces brown mushrooms, thinly sliced	1 bell pepper, seeded and thinly sliced
1 ripe tomato, seeded and chopped	1 habanero pepper, minced
Sea salt and ground black pepper, to taste	2 russet potatoes, chopped
1/2 teaspoon cayenne pepper	1 cup water
1 cup shallots, chopped	2 bay leaves
2 garlic cloves, minced	2 tablespoons olive oil
1 celery with leaves, chopped	1 cup vegetable stock
	2 tablespoons corn flour, plus 3 tablespoons of water
	1/2 teaspoon Hungarian paprika

DIRECTIONS and Cooking Time: 45 Minutes
Press the "Sauté" button to heat up the Electric Pressure Cooker. Then, heat the olive oil and sauté the shallot, garlic, potatoes, and celery until they are softened; add a splash of vegetable stock, if needed. Stir in the mushrooms, water, stock, paprika, cayenne pepper, bay leaves, and tomatoes. Secure the lid. Select the "Meat/Stew" setting; cook for 35 minutes at High pressure. Once cooking is complete, use a quick pressure release; carefully remove the lid. Make the slurry by whisking the corn flour with 3 tablespoons of water. Add the slurry back to the Electric Pressure Cooker and press the "Sauté" button one more time. Allow it to cook until the liquid has thickened. Discard bay leaves and serve warm.

Traditional Provençal Ratatouille

INGREDIENTS for Servings: 4

3 sweet peppers, seeded and sliced	1 tablespoon sea salt
	4 tablespoons extra-virgin olive oil
1 teaspoon basil	1 pound eggplant, sliced
1 teaspoon rosemary	2 onions, sliced
1 pound tomatoes, pureed	4 cloves garlic, pressed
4 tablespoons Pinot Noir	Sea salt and ground red pepper, to taste
1 cup vegetable broth	
1 teaspoon oregano	
1 pound zucchini, sliced	

DIRECTIONS and Cooking Time: 40 Minutes
Toss the eggplant with 1 teaspoon of salt in a colander. Let it sit for 30 minutes; then squeeze out the excess liquid. Transfer the eggplant to the inner pot of your Electric Pressure Cooker. Add the other ingredients to the inner pot Secure the lid. Choose the "Manual" mode and cook for 6 minutes at High pressure. Once cooking is complete, use a quick pressure release; carefully remove the lid. Season to taste with salt and pepper and serve warm. Enjoy!

Quinoa Mushroom Salad

INGREDIENTS for Servings: 4

½ cup quinoa, rinsed	½ cup green onions
¾ cup water	1 tablespoon vegetable oil
¼ teaspoon salt	1 tablespoon freshly grated ginger
½ carrot, peeled and shredded	1 tablespoon sesame oil
½ cup cremini mushrooms, diced	A pinch of red pepper flakes
1 tablespoon lime juice	

DIRECTIONS and Cooking Time: 1 Minute
Add the quinoa, salt, and water to the Electric Pressure Cooker. Secure the lid and select the "Manual" function with high pressure for 1 minute. After the beep, do a quick release and remove the lid. Meanwhile, add the remaining ingredients to a bowl and mix them well. Add the cooked quinoa to the prepared mixture and mix well. Serve as a salad.

Mushroom Pâté

INGREDIENTS for Servings: 8

½ cup grape juice	Salt and black pepper to taste
2 onions, sliced	1 cup dry Porcini mushrooms
1 ½ lb Portobello mushrooms	3 tbsps butter
1 ½ cups boiling water	

DIRECTIONS and Cooking Time: 35 Minutes
Combine dried mushrooms and boiling water in a heatproof cup. Cover and set aside. The mushrooms will soak up the water. Melt butter on Sauté. Add in onions and cook for 3 minutes until soft. Slice Portobello mushroom and add to the pot; sauté them

until golden brown, for about 4 minutes. Pour in grape juice and let it fully evaporate. Stir in the soaked mushrooms and adjust the seasoning. Seal the lid, select Manual and cook for 10 minutes at High. Do a quick release. To prepare the paté, blend the ingredients with an immersion blender, for about 5 minutes. Serve chilled.

Electric Pressure Cooker Huevos Rancheros

INGREDIENTS for Servings: 8

1 tablespoon butter	1 clove of garlic, crushed
10 eggs, beaten	1 can green chilies, drained
1 cup light cream	8 tortillas
8 ounces Mexican blend cheese, grated	1 can red enchilada sauce
½ teaspoon pepper	
¼ teaspoon chili powder	

DIRECTIONS and Cooking Time: 15 Minutes
Grease the inside of the Electric Pressure Cooker with butter. In a large bowl, mix together the eggs, cream, Mexican cheese, pepper, and chili powder. Stir in the garlic and chilies. Pour into the Electric Pressure Cooker and close the lid. Press the Manual button and adjusts the cooking time to 15 minutes. Do natural pressure release. Assemble the dish by spooning the egg casserole to tortillas and serving with enchilada sauce.

Orange Marmalade Oatmeal

INGREDIENTS for Servings: 4

2 cups old-fashioned oats	¼ cup sugar
2 ¼ cups water	2 tablespoons plain low-fat Greek yogurt
2 ¼ cups milk	2 tablespoons orange marmalade
½ teaspoon salt	Orange and kiwi slices garnish
½ teaspoon ground cinnamon	

DIRECTIONS and Cooking Time: 6 Minutes
Add all the ingredients except the garnish to the Electric Pressure Cooker. Secure the lid of the cooker and press the "Manual" function key. Adjust the time to 6 minutes and cook at high pressure. After the beep, release the pressure naturally and remove the lid. Stir the prepared oatmeal and serve in a bowl. Garnish with orange and kiwi slices on top.

Scrambled Eggs With Cranberries & Mint

INGREDIENTS for Servings: 2

4 large eggs, beaten	1 tbsp skim milk
¼ tsp cranberry extract, sugar-free	4-5 cranberries, to garnish
2 tbsp butter	Fresh mint, to garnish
¼ tsp salt	

DIRECTIONS and Cooking Time: 10 Minutes
In a bowl, whisk eggs, cranberry extract, salt, and milk. Melt butter on Sauté. Pour the egg mixture and pull the eggs across the pot with a spatula. Do not stir constantly. Cook for 2 minutes, or until thickened and no visible liquid egg lumps. When done, press Cancel and transfer to a serving plate. Top with cranberries and garnish with fresh mint.

Broccoli With Italian-style Mayonnaise

INGREDIENTS for Servings: 4

1 pound broccoli florets	3 garlic cloves, smashed
Kosher salt and ground black pepper, to taste	1/2 cup mayonnaise
	1 tablespoon Italian seasoning mix

DIRECTIONS and Cooking Time: 10 Minutes
Add 1 cup of water and steamer basket to the inner pot. Place the broccoli florets in the steamer basket. Secure the lid. Choose the "Manual" mode and cook for 1 minute at High pressure. Once cooking is complete, use a quick pressure release; carefully remove the lid. Sprinkle the garlic, salt, and black pepper over the cooked broccoli florets. Mix the mayonnaise with the Italian seasoning mix; serve your broccoli with the Italian mayo on the side. Bon appétit!

Chicken Sandwiches With Bbq Sauce

INGREDIENTS for Servings: 2-4

4 chicken thighs, boneless and skinless	2 tbsp minced fresh parsley
Salt to taste	1 tbsp lemon juice
2 cups barbecue sauce	1 tbsp mayonnaise
1 onion, minced	1½ cups iceberg lettuce, shredded
2 garlic cloves, minced	4 burger buns

DIRECTIONS and Cooking Time: 45 Minutes
Season the chicken with salt, and transfer into the pot. Add in garlic, onion and barbeque sauce. Coat the chicken by turning in the sauce. Seal the lid and cook on High Pressure for 15 minutes. Do a natural release for 10 minutes. Use two forks to shred the chicken and mix into the sauce. Press Keep Warm and let the mixture to simmer for 15 minutes to thicken the sauce, until desired consistency. In a bowl, mix lemon juice, mayonnaise, salt, and parsley; toss lettuce into the mixture to coat. Separate the chicken in equal parts to match the sandwich buns; apply lettuce for topping and complete the sandwiches.

Grapefruit Potatoes With Walnuts

INGREDIENTS for Servings: 6

12 small potatoes, chopped	2 tbsp olive oil
¾ cup walnuts, chopped	¼ tsp turmeric powder
1 cup mayonnaise	Salt and black pepper to taste
Juice of 1 lemon	1 grapefruit, chopped

DIRECTIONS and Cooking Time: 20 Minutes
Place potato chunks inside your IP and add enough water to cover them. Seal the lid, select Manual, and cook at High for 10 minutes. Quick release the pressure, and drain the potatoes. Add grapefruit and walnuts. Whisk the remaining ingredients in a bowl, and pour over the potatoes.

Vegetable Frittata With Cheddar & Ricotta

INGREDIENTS for Servings: 2-4

4 eggs	1 cup chopped broccoli, pre-cooked
8 oz spinach, finely chopped	4 tbsp olive oil
½ cup cheddar cheese	½ tsp salt
½ cup fresh ricotta cheese	¼ tsp black pepper
3 cherry tomatoes, halved	¼ tsp dried oregano
¼ cup red bell pepper, chopped	½ cup fresh celery leaves, finely chopped

DIRECTIONS and Cooking Time: 30 Minutes
Heat olive oil on Sauté. Add spinach and cook for 5 minutes, stirring occasionally. Add tomatoes, peppers, and broccoli. Cook for more 3-4 minutes. In a bowl, Whisk 2 eggs, cheddar, and ricotta. Pour in the pot and cook for 2 more minutes. Then, crack the remaining 2 eggs and cook for another 5 minutes. When done, Press Cancel. Serve immediately with chopped celery leaves.

Warm Spinach Salad With Eggs & Nuts

INGREDIENTS for Servings: 4

1 lb spinach, rinsed, chopped	1 tbsp peanuts, crushed
3 tbsp olive oil	4 eggs
1 tbsp butter	½ tsp chili flakes
1 tbsp almonds, crushed	½ tsp salt

DIRECTIONS and Cooking Time: 25 Minutes
Pour 1 ½ cups of water into the inner pot and insert a steamer basket. Place the eggs onto the basket. Seal the lid and cook on High Pressure for 5 minutes. Do a quick release. Remove the eggs to an ice bath. Wipe the pot clean, and heat oil on Sauté. Add spinach and cook for 2-3 minutes, stirring occasionally. Stir in 1 tbsp of butter and Season with salt and chili flakes. Mix well and cook for 1 more minute. Press Cancel and sprinkle with nuts. Peel and slice each egg in half, lengthwise. Transfer to a serving plate and pour over spinach mixture.

Tasty Onion Frittata With Bell Pepper

INGREDIENTS for Servings: 2

3 eggs	¼ tsp garlic powder
¼ cup bell pepper, diced	Salt and black pepper to taste
¼ cup onions, diced	A pinch of ginger powder
2 tbsp milk	

DIRECTIONS and Cooking Time: 20 Minutes
Pour 1 cup water into the pressure cooker and lower a trivet. Grease a small baking dish with cooking spray. In a bowl, beat eggs along with milk, ginger, sal, black pepper and garlic powder. Add onions and bell pepper and stir well to combine. Pour the mixture into the greased baking dish and place it on the trivet. Seal the lid, select Manual, and cook for 8 minutes at High. After the timer goes off, release the pressure quickly.

Vegan Baked Beans

INGREDIENTS for Servings: 6

1 ½ pounds pinto beans, rinsed and drained	2 onions, chopped
	1 cup molasses
8 cups water	1 cup ketchup
2 tablespoons olive oil	1 teaspoon salt
5 cloves garlic, minced	2 tablespoons soy sauce
	1 tablespoon Cholula hot sauce

DIRECTIONS and Cooking Time: 1 Hour 10 Minutes
Place the beans and water in your Electric Pressure Cooker. Secure the lid. Choose the "Bean/Chili" mode and cook for 40 minutes at High pressure. Once cooking is complete, use a natural pressure release for 10 minutes; carefully remove the lid. Set aside. Press the "Sauté" button and heat the oil until sizzling. Now, cook the onion and garlic until tender and fragrant. Add the reserved beans back to the inner pot. Stir in the remaining ingredients. Secure the lid. Choose the "Manual" mode and cook for 10 minutes at High pressure. Once cooking is complete, use a quick pressure release. Bon appétit!

Tasty Asparagus Soup

INGREDIENTS for Servings: 4

2 lb fresh asparagus, trimmed	2 tbsp butter
	1 tbsp vegetable oil
2 onions, chopped	½ tsp salt

1 cup heavy cream	½ tsp dried oregano
4 cups vegetable broth	½ tsp paprika

DIRECTIONS and Cooking Time: 40 Minutes
Melt butter on Sauté, and add 1 tbsp of oil. Stir-fry the onions for 2 minutes, until translucent. Add asparagus, oregano, salt, and paprika. Stir well and cook until asparagus soften, for a few minutes. Pour the broth and mix well to combine. Seal the lid and cook on Soup/Broth for 20 minutes on High. Do a quick release and whisk in 1 cup of heavy cream. Serve chilled or warm.

Eggplant With Steamed Eggs And Tomatoes

INGREDIENTS for Servings: 4

4 eggs	1 red bell pepper, chopped
1 pound eggplant, peeled and cut pieces	2 ripe tomatoes, chopped
1 jalapeño pepper, minced	Sea salt, to taste
2 tablespoons butter, at room temperature	2 garlic cloves, smashed
1/2 cup scallions, chopped	1/2 teaspoon freshly ground black pepper
2 teaspoons salt	

DIRECTIONS and Cooking Time: 50 Minutes
Toss the eggplant with the salt and allow it to sit for 30 minutes; then, drain and rinse the eggplant. Press the "Sauté" button to heat up the Electric Pressure Cooker. Once hot, melt the butter. Stir in the eggplant and cook for 3 to 5 minutes, stirring periodically. Add the garlic, scallions, peppers, and tomatoes; cook an additional 4 minutes. Season with salt and pepper. Secure the lid. Select the "Manual" setting; cook for 8 minutes at HIGH pressure. Once cooking is complete, use a quick release; carefully remove the lid. Reserve. Add 1 cup of water and metal rack to the Electric Pressure Cooker. Crack the eggs into ramekins; lower the ramekins onto the rack. Secure the lid. Select the "Steam" setting; cook for 5 minutes under High pressure. Serve with the eggplant mixture on the side. Bon appétit!

French Balsamic Peppers

INGREDIENTS for Servings: 2

2 tablespoons olive oil	Sea salt and ground black pepper, to taste
4 bell peppers, seeded and sliced	1/2 cup water
1/2 cup court bouillon	2 tablespoons balsamic vinegar

DIRECTIONS and Cooking Time: 10 Minutes
Press the "Sauté" button and heat the oil. Once hot, cook the peppers until just tender and fragrant. Add the salt and black pepper. Pour in the bouillon and water. Secure the lid. Choose the "Manual" mode and cook for 3 minutes at High pressure. Once cooking is complete, use a quick pressure release. Drizzle balsamic vinegar over your peppers and serve immediately.

Light & Fruity Yogurt

INGREDIENTS for Servings: 12

1 pound hulled and halved raspberries	3 tbsp gelatin
	8 cups milk
1 cup sugar	¼ cup Greek yogurt containing active cultures
1 tbsp fresh orange juice	

DIRECTIONS and Cooking Time: 24 hours
In a bowl, mash raspberries with a potato masher. Add sugar and stir well to dissolve; let soak for 30 minutes at room temperature. Add in orange juice and gelatin and mix well until dissolved. Remove the mixture and place in a sealable container, close, and allow to sit for 12 hrs to 24 hrs at room temperature before placing in a refrigerator. Refrigerate for a maximum of 2 weeks. Into the cooker, add milk and close the lid. The steam vent should be set to Venting then to Sealing. Select Yogurt until "Boil" is displayed on the readings. When complete there will be a display of "Yogurt" on the screen. Open the lid and using a food thermometer ensure the milk temperature is at least 185°F. Transfer the steel pot to a wire rack and allow cool for 30 minutes until the milk has reached 110°F. In a bowl, mix ½ cup warm milk and yogurt. Transfer the mixture into the remaining warm milk and stir without having to scrape the steel pot's bottom. Take the pot back to the base of the pot and seal the lid. Select Yogurt mode and cook for 8 hrs. Allow the yogurt to chill in a refrigerator for 1-2 hrs. Transfer the chilled yogurt to a large bowl and stir in fresh raspberry jam.

Chili Deviled Eggs

INGREDIENTS for Servings: 2

1 cup water	Salt and black pepper to taste
4 large eggs	1/8 tsp chili powder
1 tbsp cream cheese	
1 tbsp mayonnaise	

DIRECTIONS and Cooking Time: 20 Minutes
Add water, insert the steamer basket and lay the eggs inside Seal the lid and cook on High Pressure for 5 minutes. Release the Pressure quickly. Drop eggs into an ice bath to cool for 5 minutes. Peel eggs and halve them. Transfer yolks to a bowl and use a fork to mash; Stir in cream cheese, and mayonnaise. Add pepper and salt for seasoning. Ladle yolk mixture into egg white halves.

Steamed Artichoke

INGREDIENTS for Servings: 4

½ tablespoon peppercorns, whole 1 ½ garlic cloves, chopped ½ tablespoons olive oil 2 cups water	4 artichokes, trimmed 2 lemons, one juiced and one sliced Salt and pepper to taste

DIRECTIONS and Cooking Time: 10 Minutes
Pour the water and peppercorns into the insert of the Electric Pressure Cooker. Place the steamer trivet inside. Arrange the artichokes over the trivet. Secure the lid and select the "Manual" function with low pressure for 5 minutes. After the beep, do a Natural release and remove the lid. Strain the artichokes and return them back to the pot. Add the oil and all the remaining ingredients back into the Electric Pressure Cooker, and then "Sauté" for 5 minutes while stirring. Serve hot.

Morning Frittatas
INGREDIENTS for Servings: 2

3 eggs 2 tablespoons almond milk Salt and pepper, to taste ¼ cup cheddar cheese 1 tablespoon oil	1 cup water ¼ cup red bell pepper, chopped ¼ cup onion, chopped 3 silicon baking molds

DIRECTIONS and Cooking Time: 5 Minutes
Add 1 cup of water to the Electric Pressure Cooker and place the trivet inside. Add the eggs, milk, all the vegetables, spices, and cheese in a dish and mix them well. Now grease the silicon baking molds with oil and pure the mixture into each mold. Place the silicon baking molds over the trivet. Secure the lid of the cooker and press the "Manual" function key. Adjust the time to 5 minutes and cook at high pressure. After the beep, release the pressure naturally and remove the lid. Remove the stuffed molds and serve immediately.

Garlic Eggs
INGREDIENTS for Servings: 4

1 tablespoon olive oil 1 teaspoon garlic minced)1 teaspoon turmeric powder	6 small tomatoes. 4 eggs 1 green onion chopped)Salt and pepper to taste.

DIRECTIONS and Cooking Time: 15 Minutes
First, cut all the tomatoes in half or into three to four slices. Set them aside. Pour one tablespoon of olive oil into the Electric Pressure Cooker and Select "Sauté." Now add the sliced tomatoes and sauté them with their cut side down.4. Add the minced garlic and powdered turmeric into the pot. Add 4 eggs to the pot and stir them using a spatula. Scramble the eggs and mix them well with garlic, turmeric, salt and pepper. After cooking the egg scramble for 15 minutes on "Sauté" press "Cancel. Sprinkle the chopped green onions on top and serve.

Squash Tart Oatmeal
INGREDIENTS for Servings: 2-4

3 ½ cups coconut milk 1 cup steel-cut oats 1 cup shredded butternut squash ½ cup sultanas ⅓ cup honey 1 tsp ground cinnamon	¾ tsp ground ginger ½ tsp salt ½ tsp orange zest ¼ tsp ground nutmeg ¼ cup toasted walnuts, chopped ½ tsp vanilla extract

DIRECTIONS and Cooking Time: 35 Minutes
In the cooker, mix sultanas, orange zest, ginger, milk, honey, squash, salt, oats, and nutmeg. Seal the lid and cook on High Pressure for 12 minutes. Do a natural release for 10 minutes. Into the oatmeal, stir in the vanilla extract and sugar. Top with walnuts and serve.

Eggs Mushroom Casserole
INGREDIENTS for Servings: 3

3 eggs 1 cup water ½ small onion chopped ½ cup cooked ham or bacon ¼ cup heavy cream	½ cup cheddar cheese shredded ½ cup cremini mushrooms, cooked and sliced Sea salt and pepper, to taste

DIRECTIONS and Cooking Time: 10 Minutes
Add 1 cup of water to the Electric Pressure Cooker and place the trivet inside. Add all the ingredients to a bowl except the cheese and whisk well. Take a heatproof container and pour the egg mixture into it. Place the container over the trivet. Secure the lid of the cooker and press the "Manual" function key. Adjust the time to 10 minutes and cook at high pressure. After the beep, release the pressure naturally and remove the lid. Drizzle the shredded cheese on top and serve hot.

Vegetables With Halloumi Cheese
INGREDIENTS for Servings: 4

2 rosemary sprigs, leaves picked 1 thyme sprig, leaves picked 8 ounces Halloumi cheese, cubed 1/2 cup Kalamata olives, pitted and halved 1/2 cup dry Greek	1 tablespoon butter 1 teaspoon dried basil 2 tomatoes, chopped 1/3 cup water 1/2 pound eggplant, sliced 1/2 pound zucchini, sliced 2 garlic cloves, minced 1/2 cup shallots,

wine 12 ounces button mushrooms, thinly sliced 1 pepperoncini pepper, minced	chopped 1 tablespoon olive oil

DIRECTIONS and Cooking Time: 10 Minutes
Press the "Sauté" button to heat up your Electric Pressure Cooker; heat the olive oil and butter. Cook the garlic and shallots for 1 to 2 minutes, stirring occasionally. Stir in the mushrooms, pepper, eggplant, and zucchini and continue to sauté an additional 2 to 3 minutes. After that, add the basil, rosemary, thyme, tomatoes, water, and wine. Secure the lid. Choose the "Manual" mode and Low pressure; cook for 3 minutes. Once cooking is complete, use a quick pressure release; carefully remove the lid. Garnish each serving with the cheese and olives; serve warm or at room temperature.

Egg Caprese Breakfast

INGREDIENTS for Servings: 2

1 ½ cups water 2 tbsp shredded mozzarella cheese 2 cherry tomatoes, halved	2 thin slices ham 1 tsp dried basil Salt and black pepper to taste

DIRECTIONS and Cooking Time: 15 Minutes
Pour water into inner pot and fit in a trivet. Line 2 medium ramekins with a slice of ham each, crack in an egg into each and divide mozzarella, basil, and tomatoes on top. Season with salt, black pepper, and cover with foil. Place ramekins on trivet. Seal the lid, select Manual/Pressure Cook on High, and set cooking time to 3 minutes. After cooking, perform a quick pressure release to let out steam. Unlock the lid, remove bowls, and serve immediately.

Lazy Steel Cut Oats With Coconut Milk

INGREDIENTS for Servings: 2

1 tsp coconut oil 1 cup steel-cut oats 1 ½ cups water	¾ cup coconut milk Salt, to taste

DIRECTIONS and Cooking Time: 18 Minutes
Warm coconut oil on Sauté, until foaming. Add oats and cook as you stir until soft and toasted. Press Cancel. Add milk, salt and water and stir. Seal the lid, and Press Porridge. Cook for 12 minutes on High Pressure. Set steam vent to Venting to release the pressure quickly. Open the lid. Add oats as you stir to mix any extra liquid.

Braised Collard Greens With Bacon

INGREDIENTS for Servings: 4

2 ½ pounds fresh collard greens 4 garlic cloves, chopped 2 cups chicken broth Kosher salt and ground black pepper, to taste	1/4 cup dry white wine 1 onion, chopped 6 smoked bacon slices, chopped 1 teaspoon paprika 1 bay leaf

DIRECTIONS and Cooking Time: 10 Minutes
Press the "Sauté" button to preheat your Electric Pressure Cooker. Then, cook the bacon until crisp and set aside. Add the remaining ingredients to the inner pot and stir to combine. Secure the lid. Choose the "Manual" mode and cook for 5 minutes at High pressure. Once cooking is complete, use a quick pressure release; carefully remove the lid. Serve garnished with the reserved bacon. Bon appétit!

Mediterranean Tomato Soup With Feta Cheese

INGREDIENTS for Servings: 4

1 (28-ounce) can tomatoes, crushed 1/2 cup double cream 1/2 teaspoon cayenne pepper 1 teaspoon fresh basil, chopped 1/2 cup feta cheese, cubed 2 stalks green garlic, chopped 1 celery stalk, diced 2 carrots, diced	1 cup green onions, chopped 1 teaspoon fresh rosemary, chopped 1 tablespoon olive oil 2 cups vegetable broth 1 tablespoon olive oil Sea salt and ground black pepper, to your liking

DIRECTIONS and Cooking Time: 30 Minutes
Press the "Sauté" button and heat 1 tablespoon of olive oil. Sauté the green onions, garlic, celery, and carrots until softened. Add the vegetable broth, salt, black pepper, cayenne pepper, basil, rosemary, and tomatoes to the inner pot. Secure the lid. Choose the "Manual" mode and cook for 6 minutes at High pressure. Once cooking is complete, use a natural pressure release for 10 minutes; carefully remove the lid. Stir in the double cream and seal the lid again; let it sit for 10 minutes more. Ladle into soup bowls; garnish with feta and 1 tablespoon of olive oil. Bon appétit!

Brussel Sprouts With Onions & Apples

INGREDIENTS for Servings: 4

1 lb Brussel sprouts, shredded	1 ½ cups veggie stock
1 cup diced onions	1 tbsp canola oil
1 cup apples, chopped	Salt and black pepper to taste
1 tbsp cornstarch	¼ tsp cumin

DIRECTIONS and Cooking Time: 35 Minutes
Heat the oil on Sauté, add onions and apples, and cook for about 6-7 minutes. When softened add the rest of the ingredients, except for cornstarch. Seal the lid, and select Manual. Set the timer to 15 minutes at High. Do a quick pressure release. Whisk together the cornstarch and 2 tbsp water, and stir in the the pot's mixture. Cook on Sauté until the sauce thickens, for about 3 minutes.

Italian Stuffed Peppers With Mushroom And Sausage

INGREDIENTS for Servings: 4

1/2 pound Italian sausage, ground	1/2 teaspoon mustard seeds
4 medium-sized bell peppers, cored	1/2 teaspoon dried oregano
1/2 pound button mushrooms, roughly chopped	2 (15-ounce) cans tomatoes
3/4 cup buckwheat, soaked overnight	1 onion, chopped
	1 ½ cups chicken broth
1/2 teaspoon red pepper flakes, crushed	Salt and ground black pepper, to taste
1 teaspoon dried basil	2 cloves garlic, minced

DIRECTIONS and Cooking Time: 25 Minutes
Press the "Sauté" button to preheat the Electric Pressure Cooker. Once hot, add olive oil; now, sauté the onion and garlic until tender and aromatic. Add the Italian sausage and mushrooms; continue to cook an additional 2 minutes; reserve the sausage/mushroom mixture. Now, add the soaked buckwheat and chicken broth. Secure the lid. Choose the "Manual" mode and High pressure; cook for 3 minutes. Once cooking is complete, use a natural pressure release; carefully remove the lid. Add the reserved sausage/mushroom mixture and seasonings; stir to combine well. Stuff the peppers. Wipe down the Electric Pressure Cooker with a damp cloth. Add 1 ½ cups of water and metal rack to the Electric Pressure Cooker. Place the stuffed peppers in a casserole dish; add tomatoes, mustard seeds, and bay leaf. Lower the dish onto the rack. Secure the lid. Choose the "Manual" mode and High pressure; cook for 10 minutes. Once cooking is complete, use a natural pressure release; carefully remove the lid. Serve warm and enjoy!

Bacon And Cheese Crustless Quiche

INGREDIENTS for Servings: 6

6 eggs, lightly beaten	2 cups Monterey Jack cheese, grated
1 cup milk	1 cup bacon, cooked and crumbled
Salt and pepper to taste	

DIRECTIONS and Cooking Time: 10 Minutes
Spray the inner pot of the Electric Pressure Cooker with cooking spray. In a mixing bowl, mix together the eggs, milk, salt, and pepper until well-combined. Place the bacon and cheese in the Electric Pressure Cooker and pour over the egg mixture. Close the lid and press the Manual button. Adjust the cooking time to 10 minutes. Do natural pressure release.

Green Soup With Navy & Pinto Beans

INGREDIENTS for Servings: 5

1 tbsp olive oil	1 onion, chopped
2 cloves garlic, minced	3 carrots, chopped
5 cups vegetable broth	1 large celery stalk, chopped
½ cup pinto beans, soaked overnight	1 tsp dried thyme
½ cup navy beans, soaked overnight	16 oz zucchini noodles
	Salt and black pepper, to taste

DIRECTIONS and Cooking Time: 35 Minutes
Warm oil on Sauté. Stir in garlic and onion and cook for 5 minutes. Mix in pepper, broth, carrots, salt, celery, beans, and thyme. Seal the lid and cook for 15 minutes on High Pressure. Release the pressure naturally. Mix zucchini noodles into the soup and stir until wilted. Taste and adjust the seasoning.

Effortless Tomato-lentil Soup

INGREDIENTS for Servings: 4

2 cups red lentils, soaked overnight	3 tbsp tomato paste
1 carrot, cut into thin slices	2 tomatoes, wedged
	1 onion, diced
3 garlic cloves, crushed	½ tsp dried thyme, ground
	½ tsp cumin, ground
4 cups vegetable broth	Salt and black pepper to taste

DIRECTIONS and Cooking Time: 17 Minutes
Add all ingredients to the pot. Seal the lid and cook on High pressure for 7 minutes. Do a quick release.

Spinach Hash

INGREDIENTS for Servings: 3

6 eggs 1 medium green pepper, stemmed, cored, and chopped 1 cup 1 medium red pepper, stemmed, cored, and chopped 1 cup ¼ teaspoon black pepper 2 large sweet potatoes, diced	1 small onion, chopped 3 bacon strips, chopped ½ cup cheddar cheese shredded 8 oz. baby spinach, chopped ¼ teaspoon salt 1 tablespoon milk inch springform pan

DIRECTIONS and Cooking Time: 20 Minutes
Add the bacon to the Electric Pressure Cooker and select the "Sauté" function to cook for 3 minutes. Transfer the crispy cooked bacon to the greased "spring pan." Add the sweet potatoes, onion, bell peppers and spinach on top of bacon. Crack all the eggs in a bowl and whisk them well with the milk. Pour the eggs mixture over the bell peppers in the spring pan. Sprinkle salt and pepper on top and cover with aluminum foil. Pour some water into the Electric Pressure Cooker, set the trivet inside, and then place the covered spring pan over the trivet. Press the "Manual" key, adjust its settings to High pressure for 20 minutes. After it is done, do a Natural release to release the steam. Remove the lid and the spring pan. Transfer the hash to a plate. Sprinkle the shredded cheddar cheese on top and serve.

Chicken & Vegetable Rice Soup

INGREDIENTS for Servings: 4

1 lb chicken breast, boneless, skinless, cubed 1 large carrot, chopped 1 onion, chopped 1 potato, finely chopped	¼ cup rice ½ tsp salt 1 tsp cayenne pepper A handful of parsley, finely chopped 3 tbsp olive oil 4 cups chicken broth

DIRECTIONS and Cooking Time: 20 Minutes
Add all ingredients, except parsley, to the pot, and seal the lid. Cook on Soup/Broth for 15 minutes on High. Do a quick pressure release. Stir in fresh parsley and serve.

Coco Quinoa Bowl

INGREDIENTS for Servings: 3

¾ cup quinoa, soaked in water at least 1 hour 1 8 oz.) can milk, ¾ cup water A pinch of salt Toppings:	½ teaspoon cocoa powder 2 tablespoons honey Chocolate chips Whipped cream

DIRECTIONS and Cooking Time: 1o Minutes

Add all the ingredients for quinoa to the Electric Pressure Cooker. Secure the lid of the cooker and press the "Rice" function key. Adjust the time to 10 minutes and cook at low pressure. After the beep, release the pressure naturally and remove the lid. Stir the prepared quinoa well and serve in a bowl. Add the chocolate chips and whipped cream on top.

Garam Masala Parsnip & Red Onion Soup

INGREDIENTS for Servings: 4

2 tbsp vegetable oil 1 red onion, finely chopped 3 parsnips, chopped 2 garlic cloves, crushed 2 tsp garam masala ½ tsp chili powder	1 tbsp plain flour 4 cups vegetable stock 1 whole lemon, juiced Salt and black pepper to taste Strips of lemon rind, to garnish

DIRECTIONS and Cooking Time: 15 Minutes
Heat oil on Sauté, and stir-fry onion, parsnips and garlic for 5 minutes, or until soft but not changed color. Stir in garam masala and chili powder and cook for 30 seconds. Stir in flour, for another 30 seconds. Pour in the stock, lemon rind and lemon juice, and seal the lid. Cook on Manual/Pressure Cook for 5 minutes on High. Do a quick release, remove a third of the vegetable pieces with a slotted spoon and reserve. Process the remaining soup and vegetables in a food processor for about 1 minute, to a smooth puree. Return to the pot, and stir in the reserved vegetables. Press Keep Warm and heat the soup for 2 minutes until piping hot. Season with salt and pepper, then ladle into bowls. Garnish with strips of lemon, to serve.

Perfect Mediterranean Asparagus

INGREDIENTS for Servings: 4

1 lb asparagus, trimmed 1 garlic clove, minced 1 tbsp shallot, minced ½ cup chopped parsley	½ cup chopped fresh mint 2 ½ tbsp olive oil 1 tbsp lemon juice Salt and black pepper to taste

DIRECTIONS and Cooking Time: 10 Minutes
Place asparagus and pour 1 cup water in your IP. Seal the lid, and cook for 3 minutes on Manual at High. Once done, release the pressure quickly. Toss the asparagus with the remaining ingredients to combine thoroughly, and serve.

Asian Vegetable Soup

INGREDIENTS for Servings: 4

1 tablespoon light soy sauce 2 tablespoons fresh	2 carrots, trimmed and chopped Sea salt and freshly

parsley, roughly chopped	ground pepper, to taste
2 tablespoons mijiu (rice wine)	1/2 pound mushroom, sliced
1/2 teaspoon dried dill	3 cups water
1 teaspoon smoked paprika	1/2 cup milk
2 tablespoons sesame oil, softened	2 shallots, chopped
	2 cloves garlic, smashed

DIRECTIONS and Cooking Time: 15 Minutes
Press the "Sauté" button and heat the oil. Once hot, sweat the shallots and garlic until tender and translucent. Add the mushrooms and carrots. Season with salt, ground pepper, dill, and paprika. Sauté for 3 more minutes more or until the carrots have softened. Add rice wine to deglaze the pan. Add the water, milk, and light soy sauce. Secure the lid. Choose the "Manual" function, High pressure and 5 minutes. Once cooking is complete, use a quick release; carefully remove the lid. Taste, adjust the seasonings and serve in individual bowls, garnished with fresh parsley. Bon appétit!

Lentil-arugula Pancake
INGREDIENTS for Servings: 2

1 cup split yellow lentils, soaked overnight and drained	1 pinch turmeric
	¼ tsp cumin powder
	Salt to taste
2 garlic cloves, whole	3 eggs, cracked into a bowl
½ tsp smoked paprika	
¼ tsp coriander powder	1 ¼ cups water
	2 cups chopped arugula

DIRECTIONS and Cooking Time: 45 Minutes
Line a cake pan with parchment paper, grease with cooking spray, and set aside. In a blender, process lentils, garlic, paprika, turmeric, coriander, cumin, salt, eggs, and 1/3 cup of water until smooth. Pour mixture into cake pan and mix arugula through the batter. Cover with foil. Pour remaining water into the pot, fit in a trivet, and place cake pan on top. Seal the lid, select Manual/Pressure Cook on High, and set cooking time to 35 minutes. After cooking, do a quick pressure release to let out steam, and unlock the lid. Carefully remove the pan, take off foil, and release pancake onto a plate. Slice and serve with Greek yogurt.

Winter Vegetable And Lentil Stew
INGREDIENTS for Servings: 4

1 onion, chopped	2 cups brown lentils
Kosher salt and ground black pepper, to taste	1 carrot, chopped
	1 stalk celery, chopped
2 tomatoes, pureed	1 sprig rosemary, chopped
2 cups vegetable broth	
3 cloves garlic, minced	3 cups Swiss chard, torn into pieces
1 parsnip, chopped	1 tablespoon olive oil
1 sprig thyme, chopped	1 teaspoon basil

DIRECTIONS and Cooking Time: 15 Minutes
Press the "Sauté" button and heat the oil. Sauté the onion until tender and translucent or about 4 minutes. Then, stir in the garlic and cook an additional 30 seconds or until fragrant. Now, stir in the carrot, celery, parsnip, lentils, tomatoes, spices, and broth. Secure the lid. Choose the "Manual" mode. Cook for 10 minutes at High pressure. Once cooking is complete, use a quick pressure release; carefully remove the lid. Afterwards, add the Swiss chard to the inner pot. Seal the lid and allow it to wilt completely. Bon appétit!

Frittata With Vegetables & Cheese
INGREDIENTS for Servings: 4

8 oz spinach, finely chopped	4 eggs
½ cup cheddar cheese, shredded	1 cup chopped broccoli, pre-cooked
	4 tbsp olive oil
½ cup ricotta cheese, crumbled	Salt and black pepper to taste
3 cherry tomatoes, halved	¼ tsp dried oregano
¼ cup red bell pepper, chopped	½ cup fresh celery leaves, finely chopped

DIRECTIONS and Cooking Time: 30 Minutes
Heat olive oil on Sauté. Add spinach and cook for 5 minutes, stirring occasionally. Add tomatoes, peppers, and broccoli and stir-fry for 3-4 more minutes. In a bowl, Whisk eggs, cheddar cheese, and ricotta cheese. Pour in the pot and cook for 5-7 minutes. Season with salt, black pepper, and oregano; press Cancel. Serve with chopped celery leaves.

Goat Cheese & Beef Egg Scramble
INGREDIENTS for Servings: 3

6 oz lean ground beef	¼ tsp garlic powder
1 onion, chopped	¼ tsp rosemary powder
6 eggs	
¼ cup skim milk	1 tbsp tomato paste
¼ cup goat cheese	½ tsp salt
	2 tbsp olive oil

DIRECTIONS and Cooking Time: 25 Minutes
Grease the inner pot with olive oil. Stir-fry the onion, for 4 minutes, until translucent, on Sauté. Add beef and tomato paste. Cook for 5 minutes, stirring twice. Meanwhile, Whisk the eggs, milk, goat cheese, rosemary, garlic, and salt. Pour the mixture into the pot and stir slowly with a wooden spatula. Cook until slightly underdone. Remove from the heat and serve.

Delicious Chicken & Potato Soup

INGREDIENTS for Servings: 4

1 lb chicken breast, boneless, skinless, chopped	1 tsp cayenne pepper
1 onion, chopped	2 egg yolks
1 carrot, chopped	1 tsp salt
2 small potatoes, peeled, chopped	3 tbsp lemon juice
	3 tbsp olive oil
	4 cups water

DIRECTIONS and Cooking Time: 35 Minutes
Add all ingredients to the pot, and seal the lid. Set the steam release handle and cook on Soup/Broth mode for 20 minutes on High. Release the pressure naturally, for 10 minutes, open the lid and serve.

Mushroom-spinach Cream Soup

INGREDIENTS for Servings: 4

1 tbsp olive oil	1 red onion, chopped
8 button mushrooms, sliced	2 tbsp white wine
1 cup spinach, chopped	1 tbsp dry porcini mushrooms, soaked and drained
4 cups vegetable stock	Salt and black pepper to taste
2 sweet potatoes, peeled and chopped	1 cup creme fraiche

DIRECTIONS and Cooking Time: 25 Minutes
Set on Sauté and add in olive oil and mushrooms. Sauté for 3 to 5 minutes until browning on stock sides; Set aside. Add onion and spinach, and cook for 3 to 5 minutes until the onion becomes translucent. Stir in chopped mushrooms, and cook for a further 5 minutes, stirring occasionally, until golden brown. Pour in wine to deglaze the bottom of the pot, scrape to remove browned bits. Cook for 5 minutes until wine evaporates. Mix in the remaining mushrooms, potatoes, soaked mushrooms, stock, and salt. Seal the lid and cook on High Pressure for 5 minutes. Quick release the pressure. Add in pepper and creme fraiche to mix. Using an immersion blender, whizz the mixture until smooth. Stir in the Sautéed mushrooms. Add reserved mushrooms for garnish before serving.

Cheddar Baked Eggs

INGREDIENTS for Servings: 2

½ cup diced smoked kielbasa sausages	4 large eggs, cracked into a bowl
½ cup frozen hash brown potatoes	1 tbsp chopped scallions
¼ cup shredded cheddar cheese	Salt and black pepper to taste
2 cups water	

DIRECTIONS and Cooking Time: 15 Minutes
Grease a large ramekin with cooking spray and lay in ingredients in this order: sausages, hash browns, and cheddar cheese. Create a hole in the center and pour in eggs. Scatter scallions on top and season with salt and pepper. Pour water into inner pot and fit in a trivet. Place ramekin on trivet, seal the lid, select Manual/Pressure Cook on Low, and set cooking time to 2 minutes. When done, perform quick pressure release and unlock the lid. Carefully remove ramekin and serve for breakfast.

Gourmet Cilantro Salmon

INGREDIENTS for Servings: 2

2 slices smoked salmon	2 eggs
1 tsp cilantro, chopped	Salt and black pepper to taste
	1 tbsp paprika

DIRECTIONS and Cooking Time: 10 Minutes
Pour 1 cup water into the pressure cooker and lower a trivet. Grease 4 ramekins with cooking spray or olive oil. If using silicone ramekins, skip this step. Place a slice of smoked salmon at the bottom of each ramekin. Crack an egg on top of the salmon. Season with salt and pepper and sprinkle with cilantro and paprika. Arrange the ramekins on top of the trivet and seal the lid. Set Manual at High for 5 minutes. When the timer goes off, release the pressure quickly.

French Baked Eggs

INGREDIENTS for Servings: 4

Olive oil for brushing	A dash of French herb mix or any herbs of your choice
4 whole eggs	
4 slices of ham	
8 tablespoons of cream cheese	Salt and pepper to taste

DIRECTIONS and Cooking Time: 25 Minutes
Place a steam rack in the Electric Pressure Cooker and pour a cup of water. Brush 4 ramekins with olive oil and set aside. Into each ramekin, place a slice of ham, two tablespoons of cream cheese, and a dash of mixed herbs. Crack open the eggs on each of the ramekins and season with salt and pepper to taste. Place on the steam rack. Close the lid and seal the vent. Choose the Low pressure and adjust the cooking time to 25 minutes. Do natural pressure release.

Garden Vegetable Soup

INGREDIENTS for Servings: 4

1 carrot, finely chopped	½ cup celery leaves, chopped
2 spring onions, finely chopped	2 tbsp butter
1 red bell pepper, chopped, seeds removed	1 tsp vegetable oil
	4 cups vegetable broth
	1 cup milk
2 celery stalks, finely	Salt and black pepper to taste

chopped	
½ tsp dried thyme	

DIRECTIONS and Cooking Time: 22 Minutes
Melt butter on Sauté. Add carrot, onions, bell pepper, and celery. Cook for 5 minutes, stirring constantly. Pour in vegetable broth, seal the lid and cook on Manual/Pressure Cook mode for 5 minutes on High. Do a quick release. Stir in all remaining ingredients and cook for 2-3 minutes, on Sauté. Serve warm.

Green Beans Salad

INGREDIENTS for Servings: 4

½ oz. dry porcini mushrooms, soaked	1 cup water
1 lb. green beans, trimmed1 lb. potatoes, quartered	½ teaspoon sea salt, divided
	Black pepper ground to taste

DIRECTIONS and Cooking Time: 7 Minutes
Add the water, potatoes, mushrooms, and salt to the Electric Pressure Cooker. Place the steamer trivet over the potatoes. Arrange all the green beans in the steamer. Secure the lid and select the "Manual" function for 7 minutes with high pressure. After the beep, do a Natural release for 10 minutes and remove the lid. Transfer the green beans to a platter. Strain the potatoes and mushrooms. Add the potatoes and mushroom to the green beans. Mix gently, sprinkle some pepper and salt on top and serve.

Electric Pressure Cooker Bread Pudding

INGREDIENTS for Servings: 12

2 cups milk	2 egg yolks
4 whole eggs, beaten	¼ teaspoon salt
½ cup pure maple syrup	½ cup butter, melted
1 tablespoon vanilla extract	1 loaf of bread, cubed

DIRECTIONS and Cooking Time: 15 Minutes
Use a heat-proof bowl that will fit inside the Electric Pressure Cooker. Grease the bowl then set aside. Place a steamer rack in the Electric Pressure Cooker and pour in a cup of water inside the Electric Pressure Cooker. Set aside. In a blender, mix together the milk, eggs, maple syrup, vanilla, and salt. Blend for 15 seconds until smooth. Add the melted butter. Pour the custard mixture into the bowl and add the bread pieces. Press on the bread until all pieces get soaked with the custard mixture. Place on top of the steamer rack and place aluminum foil on top. Close the lid and seal the vent. Press the Steam button and adjust the cooking time to 5 minutes. Do natural pressure release. Allow to cool before eating.

Avocado Quinoa Salad

INGREDIENTS for Servings: 4

½ cup quinoa, rinsed	½ cup avocados, diced
¾ cup water	½ cup green onions
¼ teaspoon salt	1 tablespoon avocado oil
½ carrot, peeled and shredded	1 tablespoon freshly grated ginger
½ cup cabbage, chopped1 tablespoon lime juice	A pinch of red pepper flakes

DIRECTIONS and Cooking Time: 1 Minute
Add the quinoa, salt, and water to the Electric Pressure Cooker. Secure the lid and select the "Manual" function with high pressure for 1 minute. After the beep, do a quick release and remove the lid. Meanwhile, add the remaining ingredients to a bowl and mix them well. Add the cooked quinoa to the prepared mixture and mix well. Serve as a salad.

Black Bean And Egg Casserole

INGREDIENTS for Servings: 3

4 large eggs, well-beaten	½ can black beans, rinsed
½ lb. mild ground sausage	¼ cup flour
¼ large red onion, chopped	½ cup Cotija cheese*
½ red bell pepper, chopped	½ cup mozzarella cheese
¼ cup green onions	Sour cream, cilantro to garnish

DIRECTIONS and Cooking Time: 20 Minutes
Add the sausage and onion to the Electric Pressure Cooker and select the "Sauté" function and cook for 3 minutes. Combine flour with eggs and add this mixture to the sausages. Add all the vegetables, cheeses, and beans. Secure the lid of the cooker and press the "Manual" function key. Adjust the time to 20 minutes and cook at high pressure. After the beep, release the pressure naturally and remove the lid. Remove the inner pot, place a plate on top then flip the pot to transfer the casserole to the plate. Serve warm.

Meat-free Lasagna With Mushrooms

INGREDIENTS for Servings: 6

2 cloves garlic, minced	Salt and black pepper to taste
2 lb dry lasagna noodles	1 tbsp cumin
2 cups pasta sauce	2 cups mushrooms, sliced
2 cups cottage cheese	¼ cup chopped basil + some more for garnish
1 tsp red pepper flakes, crushed	

DIRECTIONS and Cooking Time: 35 Minutes

Grease a springform pan with cooking spray. Place lasagna noodles at the bottom and spread the pasta sauce evenly on top. Then place a layer of cottage cheese and sprinkle roughly with mushrooms. Season with garlic, herbs and spices and repeat the process until you run out of products. Cover with aluminum foil. Place a trivet at the bottom of your cooker, and pour 2 cups water. Place springform pan on the trivet and seal the lid. Cook for 25 minutes on Manual at High. Do a quick pressure release. Garnish with basil to serve.

Easy Homemade Omelet

INGREDIENTS for Servings: 2

2 red bell peppers, chopped	2 garlic cloves, crushed
4 eggs	1 tsp Italian seasoning mix
2 tbsp olive oil	

DIRECTIONS and Cooking Time: 20 Minutes
Grease the pot with oil. Stir-fry the peppers for 2-3 minutes on each side, or until lightly charred. Set aside. Add garlic and stir-fry for 2-3 minutes, until soft. Whisk the eggs and Season with Italian seasoning. Pour the mixture into the pot and cook for 2-3 minutes, or until set. Using a spatula, loosen the edges and gently slide onto a plate. Add grilled peppers and fold over. Serve hot.

Chickpea Hummus

INGREDIENTS for Servings: 4

½ cup dry chickpeas, soaked1 bay leaf	½ lemon, juiced
1 tablespoon olive oil	¼ teaspoon powdered cumin
2 garlic cloves	¼ teaspoon sea salt
3 cups water	¼ bunch Parsley, chopped¼ teaspoon paprika
1 tablespoon tahini	

DIRECTIONS and Cooking Time: 20 Minutes
Add 3 cups of water, chickpeas, bay leaf and garlic cloves to the Electric Pressure Cooker. Secure the lid and select the "Manual" function for 18 minutes with high pressure. After the beep, do a Natural release and remove the lid. Strain and rinse the cooked chickpeas. Discard the bay leaf. Add the oil and all the remaining ingredients to the Electric Pressure Cooker and "Sauté" for 2 minutes. Return the chickpeas to the pot and use an immerse blender to form a smooth puree. Stir and serve.

Moroccan-style Couscous Salad

INGREDIENTS for Servings: 4

1 pound couscous	1 cucumber, diced
1 tablespoon olive oil	2 cups vegetable broth
2 tablespoons sesame butter (tahini)	1/4 cup yogurt
	1 tablespoon honey
2 tablespoons fresh mint, roughly chopped	2 tomatoes, sliced
2 bell peppers, diced	A bunch of scallions, sliced

DIRECTIONS and Cooking Time: 10 Minutes
Press the "Sauté" button and heat the oil; then, sauté the peppers until tender and aromatic. Stir in the couscous and vegetable broth. Secure the lid. Choose the "Manual" mode and cook for 2 minutes at High pressure. Once cooking is complete, use a quick pressure release; carefully remove the lid. Then, stir in the remaining ingredients; stir to combine well and enjoy!

Coconut Porridge

INGREDIENTS for Servings: 2

1 cup rye flakes	2 tbsp maple syrup
A pinch of salt	¾ cup frozen black currants
1 ¼ cups coconut milk	
1 tsp vanilla extract	

DIRECTIONS and Cooking Time: 20 Minutes
In inner pot, combine rye flakes, salt, coconut milk, water, vanilla, and maple syrup. Seal the lid, select Manual/Pressure Cook on High, and set time to 5 minutes. After cooking, perform natural pressure release for 10 minutes. Stir and spoon porridge into serving bowls. Top with black currants and serve warm.

Maple-orange Glazed Root Vegetables

INGREDIENTS for Servings: 5

1 pound carrots	1 teaspoon orange peel, finely shredded
1/2 pound yellow beets	1 tablespoon maple syrup
1/2 pound red beets	Kosher salt and ground black pepper, to taste
2 tablespoons cold butter	
2 tablespoons orange juice	

DIRECTIONS and Cooking Time: 20 Minutes
Place 1 cup of water and a steamer basket in your Electric Pressure Cooker. Place the carrots and beets in the steamer basket. Secure the lid. Choose the "Steam" mode and cook for 10 minutes at High pressure. Once cooking is complete, use a quick pressure release; carefully remove the lid. Peel the carrots and beets and reserve; slice them into bite-sized pieces. Press the "Sauté" button and choose the lowest setting. Cut in butter and add the remaining ingredients. Drain the carrots and beets and add them back to the inner pot; let them cook until your vegetables are nicely coated with the glaze or about 5 minutes. Bon appétit!

Honey-mustard Glazed Cipollini Onions

INGREDIENTS for Servings: 4

3/4 cup roasted vegetable stock	2 teaspoons honey
2 bay leaves	1 rosemary sprig
1 ½ pounds Cipollini onions, outer layer eliminated	1 thyme sprig
	Sea salt and ground black pepper, to taste
1 ½ tablespoons corn starch	1 tablespoon mustard

DIRECTIONS and Cooking Time: 15 Minutes
Add all ingredients to your Electric Pressure Cooker. Secure the lid and choose the "Steam" mode. Cook for 10 minutes at High pressure. Once cooking is complete, use a quick release; carefully remove the lid. Arrange the onions on a serving platter and serve warm. Enjoy!

Fresh Red Beets

INGREDIENTS for Servings: 3

3 red beets, red part only, quartered	Salt and pepper to taste
1 cup water	

DIRECTIONS and Cooking Time: 7 Minutes
Pour a cup of water into the insert of the Electric Pressure Cooker. Place the steamer trivet inside. Arrange the beets over the trivet. Secure the lid and select the "Manual" function with high pressure for 7 minutes. After the beep, do a Natural release and remove the lid. Transfer the beets to the platter, sprinkle some salt and water on top. Serve.

Spanish Omelet

INGREDIENTS for Servings: 2

1 tbsp butter, melted	¼ cup diced yellow onion
4 oz frozen hash browns, defrosted	1 garlic clove, minced
6 large eggs	4 oz grated cheddar cheese
Salt and black pepper to taste	
1 tsp tomato paste	1 ½ cups water
¼ cup milk	

DIRECTIONS and Cooking Time: 45 Minutes
Grease a ramekin with butter and spread hash browns at the bottom. In a bowl, whisk eggs, salt, and black pepper until frothy. In another bowl, smoothly combine tomato paste with milk and mix into eggs along with onion and garlic. Pour mixture on top of hash browns. Add water to inner pot, fit in a trivet, and place ramekin on top. Seal the lid, select Manual/Pressure Cook on High, and set cooking time to 15 minutes. After cooking, perform natural pressure release for 10 minutes, then a quick pressure release to let out the remaining steam. Unlock the lid and remove ramekin. Sprinkle with cheddar cheese and place ramekin back on top of the trivet. Cover with the lid, without locking, to melt the cheese, for a minute or so. Once melted, slice and serve.

Lentil And Carrot Soup

INGREDIENTS for Servings: 4

1 cup red lentils, soaked overnight	Salt and black pepper to taste
1 red bell pepper, seeded and chopped	½ tsp cumin, ground
	2 tbsp olive oil
1 onion, peeled, chopped	A handful of parsley, to garnish
½ cup carrot puree	

DIRECTIONS and Cooking Time: 35 Minutes
Heat the oil on Sauté, add stir-fry the onion, for 4 minutes. Add the remaining ingredients and pour in 4 cups of water. Seal the lid and cook on Soup/Broth for 30 minutes on High. Do a quick Pressure release. Sprinkle with fresh parsley and serve warm.

Lime Potatoes

INGREDIENTS for Servings: 2

½ tablespoon olive oil	Freshly ground black pepper to taste
2 ½ medium potatoes, scrubbed and cubed	½ cup vegetable broth
1 tablespoon fresh rosemary, chopped	1 tablespoon fresh lemon juice

DIRECTIONS and Cooking Time: 10 Minutes
Put the oil, potatoes, pepper, and rosemary to the Electric Pressure Cooker. "Sauté" for 4 minutes with constant stirring. Add all the remaining ingredients into the Electric Pressure Cooker. Secure the lid and select the "Manual" function for 6 minutes with high pressure. Do a quick release after the beep then remove the lid. Give a gentle stir and serve warm.

Quick Mushroom-quinoa Soup

INGREDIENTS for Servings: 4

4 cups vegetable broth	1 onion, chopped
1 carrot, peeled and chopped	2 garlic cloves, smashed
1 stalk celery, diced	1 tsp salt
2 cups quinoa, rinsed	½ tsp dried thyme
1 cup mushrooms, sliced	3 tbsp butter
	½ cup heavy cream

DIRECTIONS and Cooking Time: 20 Minutes
Melt the butter on Sauté. Add onion, garlic, celery, and carrot, and cook for 8 minutes until tender. Mix in broth, thyme, quinoa, mushrooms, and salt. Seal the lid and cook on High Pressure for 10 minutes. Release pressure quickly. Stir in heavy cream. Cook for 2 minutes to obtain a creamy consistency. Serve warm.

Instant Sweet Potato

INGREDIENTS for Servings: 2

2 medium sweet potatoes, peeled Salt and pepper to taste 1 tablespoon olive oil	1 cup water 2 tablespoons chopped fresh parsley to garnish Pomegranate seeds as needed to garnish

DIRECTIONS and Cooking Time: 10 Minutes

Pour a cup of water into the insert of the Electric Pressure Cooker. Place the steamer trivet inside. Arrange the sweet potatoes over the trivet. Secure the lid and select "Steam" function for 10 minutes. After the beep, do a Natural release and remove the lid. Remove the potatoes and cut them into cubes. Add the oil and potatoes into the Electric Pressure Cooker and "Sauté" for 5 minutes while stirring. Garnish with parsley and pomegranate seeds. Serve

Strawberry Compote

INGREDIENTS for Servings: 4

2 lbs. fresh strawberries washed, trimmed, and cut in half ¼ cup sugar 2 oz. fresh orange juice	1 vanilla bean, chopped ½ teaspoon ground ginger Toast to serve with the compote

DIRECTIONS and Cooking Time: 15 Minutes

Add all the ingredients to the Electric Pressure Cooker. Secure the lid of the cooker and press the "Manual" function key. Adjust the time to 15 minutes and cook at high pressure. After the beep, release the pressure naturally and remove the lid. Stir the prepared compote, let it thicken as it cools. Serve on toast and enjoy.

Rustic Soup With Turkey Balls & Carrots

INGREDIENTS for Servings: 4

2 tbsp olive oil 6 oz turkey balls 4 cups chicken broth 1 onion, chopped 1 garlic clove, minced	3 large carrots, chopped Salt and white pepper to taste 1 tbsp cilantro, finely chopped

DIRECTIONS and Cooking Time: 35 Minutes

Heat olive oil on Sauté, and stir-fry onion, carrots and garlic for 5 minutes until soft. Add the rest of the ingredients, except for the cilantro in the pot. Seal the lid and press Manual/Pressure Cook. Cook for 25 minutes on HIgh. Release the pressure naturally for 10 minutes and serve sprinkle with cilantro.

Garam Masala Eggs

INGREDIENTS for Servings: 2

2 cups water 4 eggs, whole Ice bath 3 tsp ghee ¼ tsp fennel seeds ¼ tsp cumin seeds 4 cloves 1 tbsp cinnamon powder 3 long, red chilies, halved 1-star anise	¼ tsp ground black pepper 2 large white onions, finely chopped 2 large tomatoes, finely chopped ¼ tsp garam masala ¼ tsp turmeric powder ½ tsp chili powder Salt to taste 2 tbsp chopped cilantro leaves

DIRECTIONS and Cooking Time: 30 Minutes

Pour water in your Electric Pressure Cooker and place in eggs. Seal the lid, select Manual/Pressure Cook on High, and set time to 5 minutes. After cooking, perform a quick pressure release to let out the steam. Unlock lid and transfer eggs to an ice bath. Discard water in inner pot and wipe clean with paper towels. Peel eggs, cut in halves and set aside. Select Sauté and adjust to medium heat. Melt half of ghee and stir-fry fennel seeds, cumin, cloves, cinnamon, red chilies, and star anise, for 3 minutes or until fragrant. Add half of onions, all of tomatoes and sauté until softened, 5 minutes. Spoon mixture into a blender and process on low speed until smooth paste forms. Set aside. Melt remaining ghee in inner pot and sauté remaining onions until softened. Add the tomato paste, garam masala, turmeric powder, chili powder, and salt. Mix and cook for 3 minutes. Add eggs to coat in sauce, making sure not to break them. Allow heating for 1 to 2 minutes and spoon masala with eggs over bed rice. Garnish with cilantro and serve for lunch.

Cheesy Grits With Crispy Pancetta

INGREDIENTS for Servings: 4

3 slices pancetta, diced 1 ½ cups grated Emmental 1 cup ground grits	2 tsp butter Salt and black pepper to taste ½ cup milk

DIRECTIONS and Cooking Time: 25 Minutes

Select Sauté at High and fry the pancetta until crispy, for about 5 minutes. Set aside. Add grits, butter, milk, ½ cup water, salt, and pepper to the pot, and stir. Seal the lid and select Manual at High for 10 minutes. Once the timer has ended, do a quick pressure release again. Immediately add Emmental cheese and give the pudding a good stir. Dish the cheesy grits into serving bowls and spoon over the crisped pancetta.

Glazed Baby Carrots

INGREDIENTS for Servings: 4

1 ½ pounds baby carrots 1/4 cup champagne vinegar 3/4 cup water 3 tablespoons ghee 1/2 teaspoon ground white pepper	1/2 teaspoon paprika 2 tablespoons soy sauce 2 tablespoons sesame seeds, toasted 1/2 teaspoon kosher salt 2 teaspoons honey

DIRECTIONS and Cooking Time: 20 Minutes
Press the "Sauté" button on your Electric Pressure Cooker. Place all of the above ingredients, except for the carrots and sesame seeds, in your Electric Pressure Cooker. Cook this mixture for 1 minute, stirring frequently. Stir in baby carrots. Secure the lid. Select the "Steam" setting; cook for 10 minutes at High pressure. Once cooking is complete, use a quick pressure release; carefully remove the lid. Press the "Sauté" button one more time. Let it simmer until the sauce has reduced and thickened. Sprinkle with sesame seeds and serve at room temperature. Enjoy!

Goat Cheese & Beef Steak Salad
INGREDIENTS for Servings: 4

1 lb rib-eye steak, boneless 4 oz fresh arugula 1 large tomato, sliced ¼ cup fresh goat's cheese 4 almonds	4 walnuts 4 hazelnuts 3 tbsp olive oil 2 cups beef broth 2 tbsp red wine vinegar 1 tbsp Italian seasoning mix

DIRECTIONS and Cooking Time: 60 Minutes

Whisk together vinegar, Italian mix, and olive oil. Brush each steak with this mixture and place in your Electric Pressure Cooker. Pour in the broth and seal the lid. Cook on Meat/Stew for 25 minutes on High Pressure. Release the Pressure naturally, for about 10 minutes, and remove the steaks along with the broth. Grease the inner pot with oil and hit Sauté. Brown the steaks on both sides for 5-6 minutes. Remove from the pot and chill for 5 minutes before slicing. In a bowl, mix arugula, tomato, cheese, almonds, walnuts, and hazelnuts. Top with steaks and drizzle with red wine mixture.

Breakfast Cobbler
INGREDIENTS for Servings: 2

2 tbsps. honey ¼ cup shredded coconut 1 plum, pitted and chopped	3 tbsps. coconut oil, divided 1 apple, cored and chopped

DIRECTIONS and Cooking Time: 15 Minutes
In the Electric Pressure Cooker, combine the plum with apple, half of the coconut oil, and honey, and blend well. Lock the lid. Select the Manual mode and cook for 10 minutes at High Pressure. Once cooking is complete, do a quick pressure release. Carefully open the lid. Transfer the mixture to bowls and clean your Electric Pressure Cooker. Set your Electric Pressure Cooker to Sauté and heat the remaining coconut oil. Add the coconut, stir, and toast for 5 minutes. Sprinkle the coconut over fruit mixture and serve.

SOUPS, STEWS & CHILIS RECIPES

Chicken And Kale Soup

INGREDIENTS for Servings: 8

2 cups water	Freshly ground black pepper to taste
6 celery stalks, chopped	½ teaspoon dried thyme, crushed
4 carrots, peeled and chopped	8 cups low-sodium chicken broth
2 medium onions, chopped	2 lbs cooked chicken, shredded
4 bay leaves	4 cups fresh kale, trimmed and chopped
2 tablespoons olive oil	1 teaspoon Worcestershire sauce
½ teaspoon dried oregano, crushed	

DIRECTIONS and Cooking Time: 12 Minutes
Pour the oil into the Electric Pressure Cooker and select the 'sauté' function. Add the carrot, celery and onion to the oil and sauté for 5 minutes. Now stir in the herbs, bay leaves and black pepper and cook for another minute. Pour the water and chicken broth into the pot and secure the lid. Select the 'soup' function on the control panel and cook for 4 minutes. When you hear the beep, 'quick release' the steam, then remove the lid. Stir in the kale and chicken then cook on 'sauté' for 2 minutes. Add the Worcestershire sauce, then serve hot.

Piri Piri Chicken Soup

INGREDIENTS for Servings: 4

2 chicken breasts, cubed	2 tbsp butter
1 garlic clove, minced	1/3 cup Piri Piri spicy sauce
1 sweet onion, diced	1 tsp thyme
½ cup celery, diced	1 tbsp lemon juice
3 cups chicken bone broth	Salt and black pepper to taste

DIRECTIONS and Cooking Time: 35 Minutes
Melt butter in your Electric Pressure Cooker on Sauté and cook onion, celery, and garlic for 3 minutes. Add in the chicken and Sauté for another 4-5 minutes, stirring occasionally. Pour in chicken broth, thyme, and spicy sauce and seal the lid. Select Manual and cook for 12 minutes on High pressure. When done, allow a natural release for 10 minutes, then perform a quick pressure release and unlock the lid. Adjust the taste and drizzle with the lemon juice. Ladle into bowls and serve.

Simple Clam Chowder

INGREDIENTS for Servings: 4

2 tablespoons butter	1 pound Russet potatoes, peeled and diced
1 onion, chopped	
1 garlic clove, minced	
1 stalk celery, diced	1 teaspoon cayenne pepper
1 carrot, diced	18 ounces canned clams, chopped with juice
1 cup water	
2 cups fish stock	
Sea salt and white pepper, to taste	1 cup heavy cream

DIRECTIONS and Cooking Time: 15 Minutes
Press the "Sauté" button and melt the butter; once hot, cook the onion, garlic, celery, and carrot for 3 minutes or until they have softened. Add the water, stock, salt, white pepper, potatoes, and cayenne pepper. Secure the lid. Choose the "Manual" mode and cook for 2 minutes at High pressure. Once cooking is complete, use a quick pressure release; carefully remove the lid. Press the "Sauté" button and use the lowest setting. Stir in the clams and heavy cream. Let it simmer for about 5 minutes or until everything is thoroughly heated. Bon appétit!

Spiced Sweet Potato Soup

INGREDIENTS for Servings: 6

2 chipotle peppers, minced	Salt and black pepper to taste
4 cups vegetable broth	28 oz canned sweet potatoes
1 tbsp olive oil	
1 cup yellow onions, chopped	1 tsp garlic, smashed
	½ tsp ground allspice
3 tbsp fresh cilantro, chopped	2 tbsp pumpkin seeds, toasted
½ tsp cayenne pepper	1 cup whipping cream

DIRECTIONS and Cooking Time: 25 Minutes
Warm oil in the cooker on Sauté and cook the garlic and onions until brown, for about 3-4 minutes. Add chipotle peppers, allspice, salt, cayenne pepper, and black pepper, and cook for another 2 minutes. Then, stir in the potatoes, broth, and 2 cups of water. Seal the lid, press Manual, and cook for 10 minutes at High. Once ready, do a quick pressure release. Transfer the soup to a food processor. Blend until smooth and creamy, work in batches if necessary, then pour in the whipping cream. Sprinkle with pumpkin seeds and cilantro to serve.

Jalapeño Chicken Soup With Tortilla Chips

INGREDIENTS for Servings: 6

¾ lb chicken thighs	2 cups collard greens
1 onion, chopped	1 jalapeño pepper, deseeded and chopped
2 garlic cloves, minced	
1 cup tomatoes, chopped	½ tsp dried basil
1 tbsp ginger, minced	½ tsp dried oregano
2 tbsp butter, softened	Salt and black pepper

| | to taste |
| | 6 oz tortilla chips |

DIRECTIONS and Cooking Time: 30 Minutes
Melt the butter in your Electric Pressure Cooker on Sauté. Add in the onion, ginger, garlic, and jalapeño and cook for 3 minutes. Add in chicken and Sauté for 5 minutes, stirring often. Mix in tomatoes, 6 cups of water, oregano, basil, salt, and pepper and seal the lid. Select Manual and cook for 15 minutes. Once done, allow a natural release for 15 minutes, then perform a quick pressure release and unlock the lid. Shred the chicken and discard the bones; return it to the soup Stir in collard greens and simmer for 3 minutes on Sauté. Adjust the seasoning. Serve topped with tortilla chips.

Fall Bean Chili

INGREDIENTS for Servings: 6

6 cups vegetable stock	1 carrot, chopped
1 tsp red pepper flakes, crushed	1 onion, chopped
1 cup tomatoes, chopped	½ tsp cilantro, to garnish
1 celery stick, chopped	Salt and black pepper to taste
2 cloves garlic, minced	2 ½ cups dried white beans
	1 cup potato, chopped
	3 tbsp olive oil

DIRECTIONS and Cooking Time: 30 Minutes
Heat oil and cook garlic and onion for 3 minutes on Sauté. Add in beans along with the remaining ingredients. Seal the lid, press Manual, and cook for 20 minutes at High. Once done, do a quick pressure release. Garnish with cilantro.

Bengali Parsnip Soup

INGREDIENTS for Servings: 2-4

2 tbsp vegetable oil	4 cups vegetable stock
1 red onion, finely chopped	1 whole lemon, juiced
3 parsnips, chopped	1 tsp salt
2 garlic cloves, crushed	½ tsp black pepper, ground
2 tsp garam masala	Strips of lemon rind, to garnish
½ tsp chili powder	
1 tbsp plain flour	

DIRECTIONS and Cooking Time: 15 Minutes
Heat oil on Sauté, and stir-fry onion, parsnips and garlic for 5 minutes, or until soft but not changed color. Stir in garam masala and chili powder and cook for 30 seconds. Stir in flour, for another 30 seconds. Pour in the stock, lemon rind and lemon juice, and seal the lid. Cook on Manual/Pressure Cook for 5 minutes on High. Do a quick release, remove a third of the vegetable pieces with a slotted spoon and reserve. Process the remaining soup and vegetables in a food processor for about 1 minute, to a smooth puree. Return to the pot, and stir in the reserved vegetables. Press Keep Warm and heat the soup for 2 minutes until piping hot. Season with salt and pepper, then ladle into bowls. Garnish with strips of lemon, to serve.

Quick Chicken Soup

INGREDIENTS for Servings: 4

½ cup mushrooms, chopped	2 tbsp Olive oil
½ lb Chicken Breasts	2 garlic cloves, minced
1 large Carrot, chopped	1 Green Chili Pepper, sliced
1 large Celery Stalk, chopped	Salt and black pepper to taste
1 large White onion, chopped	2 cups Chicken Broth
	2 cups Water

DIRECTIONS and Cooking Time: 20 Minutes
Warm olive oil in your Electric Pressure Cooker on Sauté. Place the carrot, celery, onion, garlic, and green chili pepper and cook for 3 minutes. Mix in chicken broth, chicken breasts, mushrooms, and water. Seal the lid, select Soup, and cook for 10 minutes on High pressure. When done, do a quick pressure release. Remove the chicken, shred it, and back it to the pot. Cook for 3 minutes on Sauté and serve.

Root Vegetable Stew

INGREDIENTS for Servings: 5

3 stalks celery, chopped	3 cloves garlic, minced
3 cups vegetable broth	3 carrots, sliced
½ tsp coriander	10 red potatoes, chopped
1/8 tsp cayenne pepper	1 rutabaga, chopped
½ tsp ground cumin	1 (15-oz) can tomatoes, diced
Salt and black pepper to taste	1 tbsp olive oil
2 onions, diced	Fresh parsley chopped

DIRECTIONS and Cooking Time: 29 Minutes
Set your IP to Sauté and heat the olive oil. Add onions, garlic, and spices. Stir to combine and cook for about 3-4 minutes. Add the remaining ingredients, except for parsley. Seal the lid, select Manual at High, and cook for 15 minutes. Do a quick release. Add to Servings bowls and top with freshly chopped parsley. Serve.

Pumpkin & Pearl Barley Soup

INGREDIENTS for Servings: 6

1 cup pearl barley, rinsed	2 fennel stalks, diced
1 lb pumpkin, cubed	1 turnip, chopped
½ cup carrots,	3 tsp olive oil
	Salt and black pepper

| chopped | to taste |
| ½ cup parsnip, chopped | ½ tsp cayenne pepper |

DIRECTIONS and Cooking Time: 30 Minutes
Mix together barley, 6 cups of water, pumpkin, fennel, carrots, parsnip, turnip, and olive oil in your pressure cooker; season with salt. Seal the lid, press Manual, and cook for 25 minutes at High. Once cooking is over, do a quick pressure release. Stir in cayenne pepper and ladle into bowls to serve.

Spicy Broccoli And Cheese Soup

INGREDIENTS for Servings: 4

4 tablespoons butter	1 pound small broccoli florets
2 cloves garlic, pressed	1/2 teaspoon chili powder
1 teaspoon shallot powder	2 cups half and half
4 cups cream of celery soup	2 cups sharp cheddar cheese, freshly grated
Sea salt and ground black pepper, to taste	2 scallions stalks, chopped

DIRECTIONS and Cooking Time: 10 Minutes
Add the butter, garlic, shallot powder, cream of celery soup, broccoli, salt, black pepper, and chili powder to the inner pot. Secure the lid. Choose the "Manual" mode and cook for 2 minutes at High pressure. Once cooking is complete, use a quick pressure release; carefully remove the lid. Stir in the half and half and cheese. Let it simmer until everything is thoroughly heated. Divide between serving bowls and serve garnished with chopped scallions. Bon appétit!

Chicken Noodle Soup

INGREDIENTS for Servings: 6

3 tbsp butter	1 tsp oregano
1 medium onion, diced	1 tsp basil, dried
3 celery stalks, diced	1 tsp thyme, dried
2 large carrots, diced	8 cups chicken broth or vegetable broth
5 cloves garlic, minced	8 oz spaghetti noodles break in half
2 cups skinless and boneless chicken breasts, cooked and cubed	2 cups spinach, chopped
	Salt and ground black pepper to taste

DIRECTIONS and Cooking Time: 30 Minutes
To preheat the Electric Pressure Cooker, select SAUTÉ. Once hot, add the butter and melt it. Add the onion, celery, carrot and a big pinch of salt. Stir and sauté for 5 minutes until they're soft. Add the garlic, oregano, basil and thyme. Stir well and sauté for 1 minute more. Add the chicken, broth and noodles. Close and lock the lid. Press the CANCEL button to reset the cooking program, then press the MANUAL button and set the cooking time for 4 minutes at HIGH pressure. When the timer beeps, use a Quick Release. Carefully unlock the lid. Add the spinach and season with salt and pepper. Stir to mix. Serve.

Cheesy Tomato Soup

INGREDIENTS for Servings: 8

3 lb tomatoes, peeled	Salt and black pepper to taste
1 carrot, diced	4 cups chicken broth
1 onion, diced	½ cup Grana Padano, grated
¼ cup fresh basil	1 tsp garlic, minced
1 cup heavy cream	
1 tbsp tomato paste	
3 tbsp butter	

DIRECTIONS and Cooking Time: 35 Minutes
Melt butter on Sauté and cook onion, celery, garlic, and carrot until soft, 5 minutes. Stir in the remaining ingredients, except for the cream and cheese. Seal the lid, select Manual, and cook for 25 minutes at High. When it goes off, do a quick pressure release. Stir in heavy cream and grated Grana Padano cheese. Serve.

Gingered Squash Soup

INGREDIENTS for Servings: 2-4

4 leeks, washed and trimmed	1 garlic clove, crushed
2 cups butternut squash, chopped	4 cups vegetable broth
	2 tbsp olive oil
¼ tsp black pepper, ground	1 tsp cumin
	1 tsp ginger powder
1 tsp sea salt	
1 tsp ginger, grated	

DIRECTIONS and Cooking Time: 35 Minutes
Stir-fry leeks and garlic for about 5 minutes, on Sauté. Add ginger powder and cumin. Give it a good stir and continue to cook for 1 more minute. Pour in the remaining ingredients and seal the lid. Cook on Soup/Broth mode for 10 minutes on High. Release the pressure naturally, for about 10 minutes.

Simple Chicken And Kale Soup

INGREDIENTS for Servings: 4

1 tbsp. coconut oil	1 onion, diced
2 celery stalks, chopped	3 cups water
	Salt and pepper, to taste
1 lb. boneless chicken breasts	4 cups chopped kale

DIRECTIONS and Cooking Time: 20 Minutes
Press the Sauté button on the Electric Pressure Cooker and heat the coconut oil. Sauté the onions and celery for 2 minutes until soft. Add the chicken breasts and sear for 2 minutes on each side or until lightly browned. Pour in the water and sprinkle salt and pepper for seasoning. Lock the lid. Set to Poultry

mode and set the timer to 15 minutes at High Pressure. When the timer goes off, do a natural pressure release for 10 minutes, then release any remaining pressure. Carefully open the lid. Press the Sauté button and add the kale. Allow to simmer for 3 minutes. Serve warm.

Rich And Easy Chicken Purloo

INGREDIENTS for Servings: 8

1 tablespoon olive oil	2 bay leaves
1 onion, chopped	1 teaspoon mustard seeds
3 pounds chicken legs, boneless and skinless	1/4 teaspoon marjoram
2 garlic cloves, minced	Seasoned salt and freshly ground black pepper, to taste
5 cups water	
2 carrots, diced	
2 celery ribs, diced	1 teaspoon cayenne pepper
	2 cups white long-grain rice

DIRECTIONS and Cooking Time: 25 Minutes
Press the "Sauté" button and heat the olive oil. Now, add the onion and chicken legs; cook until the onion is translucent or about 4 minutes. Stir in the minced garlic and continue to cook for a minute more. Add the water. Secure the lid. Choose the "Manual" mode and cook for 10 minutes at High pressure. Once cooking is complete, use a quick pressure release; carefully remove the lid. Add the remaining ingredients. Secure the lid. Choose the "Manual" mode and cook for 5 minutes at High pressure. Once cooking is complete, use a quick pressure release; carefully remove the lid. Serve warm.

Parsley Pork Chili

INGREDIENTS for Servings: 4

½ lb small pork meatballs	1 bell pepper, diced
3 potatoes, cubed	1 (14.5-oz) can tomatoes
2 cloves garlic, minced	2 tbsp olive oil
1 onion, chopped	2 tsp parsley, chopped

DIRECTIONS and Cooking Time: 30 Minutes
Press Sauté and warm oil in the IP. Cook garlic and onion for 3 minutes. Add in the remaining ingredients, except for parsley. Pour in 1 cup of water. Seal the lid, press Manual, and cook for 20 minutes at High. Once ready, do a quick pressure release. Garnish with fresh parsley to serve.

Cashew & Tomato Soup

INGREDIENTS for Servings: 4

½ ground cumin	½ tbsp dried basil
15 oz tomato puree	1 ½ tbsp quick oats
15 oz diced tomatoes	2 minced garlic cloves
4 tbsp cashew	Salt and black pepper to taste
2 cups vegetable stock	

DIRECTIONS and Cooking Time: 15 Minutes
Place the tomato puree, diced tomatoes, cashew, vegetable stock, dried basil, oats, cumin, and garlic in your Electric Pressure Cooker. Seal the lid, select Manual, and cook for 4 minutes on High pressure. When done, allow a natural release and unlock the lid. Using an immersion blender, pulse the Soup until smooth. Sprinkle with salt and pepper before serving.

"eat-me" Ham And Pea Soup

INGREDIENTS for Servings: 6

1 onion, diced	1 lb ham chunks
1 lb split peas, dried	1 ½ tsp dried sage
2 carrots, diced	Salt and black pepper to taste
2 fennel bulb, diced	

DIRECTIONS and Cooking Time: 35 Minutes
Put all ingredients in the IP and pour in 6 cups of water. Seal the lid, and select Manual at High. Cook for 20 minutes. Do a quick pressure release. Adjust the seasoning. Serve in soup bowls.

Cheesy Cauliflower Soup

INGREDIENTS for Servings: 4

1 carrot, chopped	2 tsp minced' garlic
¼ cup cream cheese	¼ cup chopped' onion
1 ½ cups cauliflower florets	Salt and black pepper to taste
1 cup vegetable broth	

DIRECTIONS and Cooking Time: 10 Minutes
Place the cauliflower florets, carrot, minced garlic, chopped onion, salt, black pepper, and vegetable broth in your Electric Pressure Cooker. Seal the lid, select Manual, and cook for 6 minutes on High pressure. When done, perform a quick pressure release and unlock the lid. Mix in cream cheese until well combined. Blend the Soup until smooth with an immersion blender. Divide between bowls and serve.

Thai Coconut Curry Stew

INGREDIENTS for Servings: 5

2 tablespoons sesame oil	1/2 cup tomato paste
2 pounds beef chuck, cubed	1 tablespoon soy sauce
2 onions, thinly sliced	1/2 teaspoon ground cloves
2 cloves garlic, pressed	1/2 teaspoon cardamom
1 (2-inch galangal piece, peeled and sliced	1/2 teaspoon cumin
	1 cinnamon quill
	Sea salt and ground white pepper, to taste
1 Bird's eye chili pepper, seeded and	1/2 (13.5-ounce can

minced	full-fat coconut milk
4 cups chicken bone broth	2 cups cauliflower florets
1/4 cup Thai red curry paste	2 tablespoons fresh cilantro, roughly chopped

DIRECTIONS and Cooking Time: 50 Minutes
Press the "Sauté" button and heat the sesame oil. When the oil starts to sizzle, cook the meat until browned on all sides. Add a splash of broth and use a spoon to scrape the brown bits from the bottom of the pot. Next, stir in the onion, garlic, galangal, chili pepper, tomato paste, broth, curry paste, soy sauce, and spices. Secure the lid. Choose the "Soup/Broth" mode and cook for 40 minutes at High pressure. Once cooking is complete, use a quick pressure release; carefully remove the lid. After that, add the coconut milk and cauliflower to the inner pot. Secure the lid. Choose the "Manual" mode and cook for 4 minutes at High pressure. Once cooking is complete, use a quick pressure release; carefully remove the lid. Serve garnished with fresh cilantro. Enjoy!

Grandma's Noodle Soup
INGREDIENTS for Servings: 6

2 tablespoons olive oil	1 bay leaf
2 carrots, diced	Salt and freshly ground black pepper
2 parsnips, diced	2 pounds chicken thighs drumettes
1 yellow onion, chopped	
2 cloves garlic, minced	2 cups wide egg noodles
6 cups chicken bone broth	1/4 cup fresh cilantro, roughly chopped

DIRECTIONS and Cooking Time: 20 Minutes
Press the "Sauté" button and heat the oil. Once hot, cook the carrots, parsnips, and onions until they are just tender. Add the minced garlic and continue to cook for a minute more. Add the chicken bone broth, bay leaf, salt, black pepper, and chicken to the inner pot. Secure the lid. Choose the "Manual" mode and cook for 9 minutes at High pressure. Once cooking is complete, use a quick pressure release; carefully remove the lid. Shred the cooked chicken and set aside. Stir in noodles and press the "Sauté" button. Cook approximately 5 minutes or until thoroughly heated. Afterwards, add the chicken back into the soup. Serve garnished with fresh cilantro. Bon appétit!

Chickpea & Spinach Chili
INGREDIENTS for Servings: 4

1 tbsp olive oil	28 oz canned tomatoes
1 onion, diced	
1 cup chickpeas, soaked, rinsed	4 cups chicken broth
	2 cups spinach, chopped

DIRECTIONS and Cooking Time: 75 Minutes
On Sauté and warm oil. Cook onion for 5 minutes. Pour in broth and chickpeas and stir. Seal the lid, press Manual, and cook for 45 minutes at High. Once done, release the pressure quickly. Stir in spinach and cook for 5 minutes until wilted, on Sauté. Serve hot.

Authentic Kentucky Burgoo
INGREDIENTS for Servings: 8

2 tablespoons lard, melted	2 cups tomato puree
	2 parsnips, sliced thickly
2 onions, chopped	
1 pound pork shank, cubed	1 celery rib, sliced thickly
2 pounds beef shank, cubed	2 sweet peppers, seeded and sliced
1 pound chicken legs	1 jalapeno pepper, seeded and minced
1/2 cup Kentucky bourbon	
	1 teaspoon dried sage, crushed
4 cups chicken broth	
2 cups dry lima beans, soaked	1 teaspoon dried basil, crushed
1 pound potatoes, diced	Salt and freshly ground black pepper, to taste
2 carrots, sliced thickly	

DIRECTIONS and Cooking Time: 1 Hour
Press the "Sauté" button and melt 1 tablespoon of lard. Once hot, sauté the onion until tender and translucent; reserve. Add the remaining tablespoon of lard; brown the meat in batches until no longer pink or about 4 minutes. Add a splash of Kentucky bourbon to deglaze the pot. Pour chicken broth into the inner pot. Secure the lid. Choose the "Meat/Stew" mode. Cook for 45 minutes at High pressure. Once cooking is complete, use a quick pressure release; carefully remove the lid. Shred chicken meat and discard the bones; add the chicken back to the inner pot. Next, stir in lima beans and tomato puree. Secure the lid. Choose the "Manual" mode. Cook for 5 minutes at High pressure. Once cooking is complete, use a quick pressure release; carefully remove the lid. Then, stir in the remaining ingredients, including the sautéed onion. Secure the lid. Choose the "Manual" mode. Cook for 5 minutes at High pressure. Once cooking is complete, use a quick pressure release; carefully remove the lid. Serve with cornbread if desired.

Veal And Buckwheat Groat Stew
INGREDIENTS for Servings: 4

¼ cup buckwheat groats	3 cups low-sodium beef stock
1 tsp. olive oil	Salt and pepper, to taste
1 onion, chopped	
7 oz. veal shoulder	

DIRECTIONS and Cooking Time: 50 Minutes
Add the buckwheat and pour in enough water to cover the buckwheat in the Electric Pressure Cooker. Stir the ingredients to combine well. Lock the lid. Press Manual. Set the timer to 12 minutes at Low Pressure. Once the timer goes off, press Cancel. Do a natural pressure release, then release any remaining pressure. Drain water and set the buckwheat aside. Press the Sauté bottom on the Electric Pressure Cooker. Add and heat the olive oil. Add the onions and cook for 3 minutes until translucent. Add the veal shoulder and sauté for 4 to 5 minutes to evenly brown. Pour in the beef stock. Sprinkle with salt and pepper. Lock the lid. Press Manual. Set the timer to 30 minutes at High Pressure. Once the timer goes off, press Cancel. Do a natural pressure release for 8 to 10 minutes. Open the lid, mix in the buckwheat and transfer them in a large bowl and serve.

Pecorino Mushroom Soup

INGREDIENTS for Servings: 4

2 cups Pecorino cheese, shredded	2 Garlic cloves
3 cups Mushrooms, chopped	2 cups Thyme, chopped
2 tbsp Butter	2 tbsp Almond flour
1 onion, chopped	3 cups Chicken stock
	Salt and black pepper to taste

DIRECTIONS and Cooking Time: 20 Minutes
Place the butter and onion in your Electric Pressure Cooker and cook for 2 minutes on Sauté. Mix in mushrooms, garlic cloves, thyme, chicken stock, almond flour, salt, and black pepper. Seal the lid, select Manual, and cook for 10 minutes on High. When done, allow a natural release for 10 minutes and unlock the lid. Serve garnished with shredded cheese.

Black Bean Soup

INGREDIENTS for Servings: 4

45 oz. canned black beans and juice	2½ cups salsa
½ cup chopped cilantro	1 garlic clove
	2 cups water
	2 tsps. ground cumin

DIRECTIONS and Cooking Time: 20 Minutes
In the Electric Pressure Cooker, mix the salsa with black beans, cilantro, garlic, water, and cumin, stir to combine well. Lock the lid. Select the Manual mode, then set the timer for 15 minutes at High Pressure. Once the timer goes off, do a quick pressure release. Carefully open the lid. Stir soup one more time, then ladle into bowls and serve.

Gingery Butternut Squash Soup

INGREDIENTS for Servings: 6

2 garlic cloves, minced	4 cups Chicken broth
1 peeled and diced Butternut Squash	1 cup Heavy cream
	2 tbsp vegetable oil
1 tbsp Ginger powder	Salt and black pepper to taste

DIRECTIONS and Cooking Time: 25 Minutes
Place the vegetable oil and half of the butternut squash cubes and cook for 5 minutes until browns on Sauté. Add in the remaining cubes, garlic, ginger powder, chicken broth, heavy cream, salt, and black pepper. Seal the lid, select Manual, and cook for 10 minutes on High pressure. When done, perform a quick pressure release and unlock the lid. Using an immersion blender, pulse until purée. Serve immediately.

Turkey & Vegetable Stew

INGREDIENTS for Servings: 6

1 cup onion, diced	2 cups baby carrots
3 cups chicken broth	2 pounds turkey thigh
3 stalks celery, chopped	2 cups russet potatoes, chopped

DIRECTIONS and Cooking Time: 25 Minutes
Place all the ingredients in your IP. Stir, seal the lid, select Manual at High, and cook for 15 minutes. Do a quick release. Serve hot.

Authentic French Onion Soup

INGREDIENTS for Servings: 4

4 tablespoons butter, melted	Kosher salt and ground white pepper, to taste
1 pound onions, thinly sliced	1 loaf French bread, sliced
1/2 teaspoon dried sage	1 cup mozzarella cheese, shredded
4 cups chicken bone broth	

DIRECTIONS and Cooking Time: 10 Minutes
Press the "Sauté" button and melt the butter. Once hot, cook the onions until golden and caramelized. Add the salt, pepper, sage, and chicken bone broth. Secure the lid. Choose the "Manual" mode and cook for 2 minutes at High pressure. Once cooking is complete, use a quick pressure release; carefully remove the lid. Divide the soup between four oven safe bowls; top with the bread and shredded cheese; now, place the bowls under the broiler for about 4 minutes or until the cheese has melted. Bon appétit!

Chicken Spinach Corn Soup

INGREDIENTS for Servings: 5

1 tablespoon olive oil	1 tablespoon fish sauce
2 medium chicken breasts, thinly sliced	2 tablespoons light

3 scallions, chopped	soy sauce
1 large white potato, peeled and diced	2 large cloves of garlic, diced
1 tablespoon green onion, chopped	⅓ teaspoon white pepper
1 tablespoon ginger, grated	1 teaspoon salt
3 cups frozen corn kernels	1 tablespoon arrowroot powder
4 cups chicken broth	3-4 handfuls of baby spinach leaves
	2 eggs

DIRECTIONS and Cooking Time: 10 Minutes
Add the oil, green onions, chicken, potato, scallions and ginger, into the Electric Pressure Cooker and stir fry on the 'sauté' function for 5 minutes. Place the corn kernels and 1 cup chicken broth into a blender. Blend well to form a smooth puree. Now put the remaining ingredients and corn mixture into the cooker and secure the lid. Cook for 5 minutes at high pressure on 'manual' function. After the beep, 'natural release' the steam and remove the lid. Switch the cooker to the 'sauté' mode. Crack the eggs into a small bowl and whisk them well. Pour the egg mix into the soup, stirring constantly. Dissolve the arrowroot powder in water and stir it into the soup. Cook for 1 minute then serve hot.

Tofu And Miso Soup

INGREDIENTS for Servings: 4

1 cup silken tofu, cubed	1 carrot, chopped
½ onion, diced	4 cups water
2 celery stalks, chopped	1 tbsp tamari sauce
	2 tbsp miso paste
	Salt to taste

DIRECTIONS and Cooking Time: 20 Minutes
Combine all of the ingredients, except for the miso and salt, in the Electric Pressure Cooker and stir to mix. Close and lock the lid. Select the POULTRY setting and set the cooking time for 7 minutes. When the timer goes off, use a Quick Release. Carefully open the lid. Whisk together the miso paste with some of the soup. Pour the mixture in the soup and stir. Season with salt. Serve.

Rice And Beef Soup

INGREDIENTS for Servings: 4-6

1 lb beef meat, ground	½ cup white rice
1 tbsp vegetable oil	15 oz canned garbanzo beans, rinsed
1 celery rib, chopped	14 oz canned tomatoes, crushed
1 yellow onion, chopped	12 oz spicy V8 juice
3 cloves garlic, minced	28 oz canned beef stock
1 potato, cubed	Salt and black pepper to taste
2 carrots, thinly sliced	½ cup frozen peas

DIRECTIONS and Cooking Time: 30 Minutes
To preheat the Electric Pressure Cooker, select SAUTÉ. Add the ground beef and cook, stirring, for 5 minutes, until browned. Transfer the meat to a bowl. Add the oil, celery and onion. Stir and sauté for 5 minutes. Add the garlic and sauté for another 1 minute. Add the potato, carrots, rice, beans, tomatoes, spicy juice, stock, browned beef, salt and pepper. Mix well. Press the CANCEL key to stop the SAUTÉ function. Close and lock the lid. Select MANUAL and cook at HIGH pressure for 5 minutes. When the timer beeps, use a Quick Release. Carefully unlock the lid. Add the peas to the pot and stir. Let it sit for 5 minutes and serve.

Ethiopian Spinach And Lentil Soup

INGREDIENTS for Servings: 6

2 tablespoons butter	¼ teaspoon cayenne pepper
1 tablespoon olive oil	¼ teaspoon cardamom powder
1 onion, finely chopped	¼ teaspoon nutmeg, grated
1 teaspoon garlic powder	2 cups lentils, soaked overnight then rinsed
2 teaspoons ground coriander	8 cups water
½ teaspoon cinnamon powder	Salt and pepper
½ teaspoon turmeric powder	2 cups spinach leaves, chopped
¼ teaspoon clove powder	4 tablespoons lemon juice

DIRECTIONS and Cooking Time: 60 Minutes
Press the Sauté button on the Electric Pressure Cooker and heat the butter and olive oil. Sauté the onion, garlic powder, coriander, cinnamon, turmeric, clove, cayenne pepper, cardamom, and nutmeg until fragrant. Add the lentils and season with salt and pepper to taste. Close the lid and press the Manual button. Adjust the cooking time to 60 minutes or until the beans are soft. Do quick pressure release. Once the lid is off, press the Sauté button and add the spinach leaves and lemon juice. Simmer until the leaves have wilted.

Ham And Potato Soup

INGREDIENTS for Servings: 4-6

2 tbsp butter	1 cup cooked ham, diced
8 cloves garlic, minced	½ cup cheddar cheese, grated
1 onion, diced	4 cups chicken broth
2 lbs Yukon Gold potatoes, cut into small chunks	Salt and ground black pepper to taste
A dash of cayenne pepper	2 tbsp fried bacon bits

DIRECTIONS and Cooking Time: 40 Minutes
To preheat the Electric Pressure Cooker, select SAUTÉ. Once hot, add the butter and melt it. Add the garlic and onion, sauté for 1-2 minutes, or until fragrant. Add the potatoes and sauté for 3 minutes more. Add the cayenne pepper, cooked ham, and cheese. Pour in the broth and stir well. Season with salt and pepper. Close and lock the lid. Press the CANCEL button to reset the cooking program, then press the MANUAL button and set the cooking time for 25 minutes at HIGH pressure. Once timer goes off, use a Quick Release. Carefully unlock the lid. Top with bacon bits and serve.

Vegan Pottage Stew

INGREDIENTS for Servings: 4

2 tablespoons olive oil	1 turnip, diced
1 onion, chopped	2 bay leaves
2 garlic cloves, minced	2 thyme sprigs
2 carrots, diced	2 rosemary sprigs
2 parsnips, diced	Kosher salt and freshly ground black pepper, to taste
4 cups vegetable broth	1/4 cup red wine
	1 cup porridge oats

DIRECTIONS and Cooking Time: 15 Minutes
Press the "Sauté" button and heat the olive oil until sizzling. Now, sauté the onion and garlic until just tender and fragrant. Add the remaining ingredients to the inner pot; stir to combine. Secure the lid. Choose the "Manual" mode and cook for 10 minutes at High pressure. Once cooking is complete, use a quick pressure release; carefully remove the lid. Ladle into individual bowls and serve immediately. Bon appétit!

Autumn Pumpkin Soup

INGREDIENTS for Servings: 2-4

1.5 lb pumpkin, pureed	1 tbsp ground turmeric
1 onion, peeled and chopped	½ tsp salt
4 cups vegetable broth	A handful of fresh parsley
½ tbsp double cream	3 tbsp olive oil

DIRECTIONS and Cooking Time: 35 Minutes
Add onion, pumpkin, turmeric, salt, and oil to your Electric Pressure Cooker. Pour in broth and stir well. Seal the lid and adjust the steam release handle. Press Soup/Broth and cook for 30 minutes on High. Do a quick release. With an immersion blender, blend until smooth. Stir in cream and top with freshly chopped parsley.

Creamy Mushroom Soup With Chicken

INGREDIENTS for Servings: 2

1 celery stalk, chopped	½ cup water
¼ cup diced mushrooms	2 tbsp diced carrots
	1 tsp minced garlic
½ lb boneless chicken breast	Salt and black pepper to taste
¼ cup heavy cream	

DIRECTIONS and Cooking Time: 20 Minutes
Slice the chicken breast into small cubes and remove them to your Electric Pressure Cooker. Add in celery, minced garlic, salt, black pepper, and water. Seal the lid, select Pressure Cook, and cook for 10 minutes on High pressure. When done, perform a quick pressure release and unlock the lid. Stir in heavy cream, mushrooms, and carrots. Seal the lid, select Manual, and cook for 3 minutes on High pressure. When done, perform a quick pressure release and unlock the lid. Divide between bowls and serve.

Green Bean Soup

INGREDIENTS for Servings: 3

½ pound lean ground beef	½ teaspoon ground cumin
½ tablespoon garlic, minced	½ pound fresh green beans, trimmed and cut into 1-inch pieces
½ tablespoon olive oil	2 cups low-sodium beef broth
½ medium onion, chopped	
1 teaspoon dried thyme, crushed	Freshly ground black pepper, to taste
1½ cups fresh tomatoes, chopped finely	⅛ cup Parmesan cheese, freshly grated

DIRECTIONS and Cooking Time: 30 Minutes
Select the 'sauté' function on your Electric Pressure Cooker. Pour in the oil, add the beef, and cook for 5 minutes. Add the thyme, cumin and garlic, then cook for 3 minutes. Now stir in the beans, tomatoes and broth and secure the lid. Set the 'manual' function to low pressure and cook for 20 minutes. 'Quick release' the steam and remove the lid. Drizzle some black pepper and Parmesan cheese on top. Serve hot.

Fast Chicken Rice Soup

INGREDIENTS for Servings: 2-4

1 lb chicken breast, boneless, skinless, cubed	¼ cup rice
	½ tsp salt
	1 tsp cayenne pepper
1 large carrot, chopped	A handful of parsley, finely chopped
1 onion, chopped	3 tbsp olive oil
	4 cups chicken broth

| 1 potato, finely chopped | |

DIRECTIONS and Cooking Time: 20 Minutes
Add all ingredients, except parsley, to the pot, and seal the lid. Cook on Soup/Broth for 15 minutes on High. Do a quick pressure release. Stir in fresh parsley and serve.

Bean And Ham Soup

INGREDIENTS for Servings: 6-8

1 leftover ham bone with meat	1 can diced tomatoes
1 lb white beans, rinsed	1 onion diced
1 clove garlic, minced	1 tsp chili powder
	1 lemon, juiced
	8 cups chicken broth

DIRECTIONS and Cooking Time: 1 Hour 10 Minutes
Combine all of the ingredients in the Electric Pressure Cooker and stir to mix. Close and lock the lid. Select the BEAN/CHILI setting and set the cooking time for 50 minutes. When the timer beeps, use a Quick Release. Let the soup sit for 10 minutes. Carefully unlock the lid. Serve.

Two-cheese Carrot Sauce

INGREDIENTS for Servings: 2-4

1 carrot, shredded	1 cup cream cheese
½ cup gorgonzola cheese	½ tsp black pepper, ground
3 cups vegetable broth	1 tsp garlic powder
1 cup gruyere cheese, crumbled	1 tbsp fresh parsley, finely chopped

DIRECTIONS and Cooking Time: 15 Minutes
Combine all ingredients in a large bowl. Pour in the Electric Pressure Cooker, Seal the lid and cook on High Pressure for 8 minutes. Do a natural release, for 10 minutes. Store for up to 5 days.

Borscht Beet Soup

INGREDIENTS for Servings: 7

2 medium white onions, chopped	½ cup dried porcini mushrooms
2 teaspoons salt	4 tablespoons apple cider vinegar
4 tablespoons olive oil	3 tablespoons tomato paste
4 large white potatoes, peeled and diced2 large carrots, grated4 medium beets½ medium white cabbage, thinly sliced8 medium cloves of garlic, diced	2 cups beef stock
	2 cups vegetable stock
	1 teaspoon pepper
	10 cups waterFresh parsley and sour cream to garnish

DIRECTIONS and Cooking Time: 15 Minutes

Put the oil and onion in the Electric Pressure Cooker and cook for 3 minutes on the 'sauté' function. Add the carrots, beets, potatoes and cabbage, and cook for 1 minute. Stir in the rest of the ingredients and secure the lid. Select the 'manual' function and cook for 10 minutes at high pressure. After the beep, 'natural release' the steam, then remove the lid. Serve hot with parsley and cream on top.

Peppery Ground Pork Soup

INGREDIENTS for Servings: 4

1 pound ground pork	2 sweet peppers, seeded and sliced
1 teaspoon Italian seasoning	1 jalapeno pepper, seeded and minced
1 teaspoon garlic powder	2 ripe tomatoes, pureed
Sea salt and ground black pepper, to taste	4 cups chicken stock

DIRECTIONS and Cooking Time: 30 Minutes
Press the "Sauté" button to preheat your Electric Pressure Cooker. Then, brown the ground pork until no longer pink or about 3 minutes. Add the remaining ingredients to the inner pot and stir. Secure the lid. Choose the "Manual" mode and cook for 10 minutes at High pressure. Once cooking is complete, use a natural pressure release for 10; carefully remove the lid. Serve warm. Bon appétit!

Old-fashioned Duck Soup With Millet

INGREDIENTS for Servings: 4

2 tablespoons olive oil	4 cups water
1 pound duck portions with bones	1/2 cup millet, rinsed
2 garlic cloves, minced	Salt and freshly cracked black pepper, to taste
1 tablespoon chicken bouillon granules	1/4 cup fresh scallions, chopped

DIRECTIONS and Cooking Time: 20 Minutes
Press the "Sauté" button and heat the oil. Once hot, brown your duck for 4 to 5 minutes; stir in the garlic and cook an additional 30 seconds or until aromatic. Add the remaining ingredients. Secure the lid. Choose the "Manual" mode and cook for 12 minutes at High pressure. Once cooking is complete, use a quick pressure release; carefully remove the lid. Remove the cooked duck to a cutting board. Shred the meat and discard the bones. Put your duck back into the inner pot. Stir and serve immediately. Bon appétit!

Thai Tom Saap Pork Ribs Soup

INGREDIENTS for Servings: 4

1 lb. pork spare ribs	Salt and pepper, to taste
4 lemongrass stalks	
10 galangal slices	

| 10 kaffir lime leaves | 1 tbsp. sesame oil |
| 6 cups water | Cilantro, to taste |

DIRECTIONS and Cooking Time: 30 Minutes
In the Electric Pressure Cooker, place the spare ribs, lemongrass, galangal, and kaffir lime leaves. Pour in the water and sprinkle salt and pepper for seasoning. Lock the lid. Set on the Manual mode, then set the timer to 30 minutes at High Pressure. When the timer goes off, do a natural pressure release, then release any remaining pressure. Carefully open the lid. Drizzle with sesame oil and garnish with cilantro before serving.

Bacon And Veggie Soup

INGREDIENTS for Servings: 3

½ tablespoon olive oil	½ green bell pepper, seeded and choppedSalt, and freshly ground black pepper to taste
½ small yellow onion, chopped	
1 garlic clove, minced	
½ head cauliflower, chopped roughly	½ cup half-and-half cream*
2 cups homemade chicken broth	3 cooked turkey bacon slices, chopped
1 cup Cheddar cheese, shredded	2 dashes hot pepper sauce

DIRECTIONS and Cooking Time: 20 Minutes
Add the oil with onion and garlic in the Electric Pressure Cooker and "Sauté" for 3 minutes Stir in the broth, salt, black pepper, cauliflower and bell pepper then secure the lid. Select the 'soup'" function and cook for 15 minutes. After the beep, 'quick release' the steam then remove the lid. Stir in the remaining ingredients and cook on the 'sauté' function for 5 minutes. Serve hot.

Hearty Beef Soup

INGREDIENTS for Servings: 6

2 tbsp olive oil	½ cup pearl barley, rinsed
2 lb beef stew meat, cubed	1 bay leaf
1 leek, finely chopped	6 cups beef bone broth
2 garlic cloves, minced	½ tsp soy sauce sauce
2 carrots, chopped	Salt and black pepper to taste
1 celery stalk, chopped	1 tbsp Parmesan cheese, grated

DIRECTIONS and Cooking Time: 1 Hour 10 Minutes
Warm the olive oil in your Electric Pressure Cooker on Sauté. Season beef with salt and pepper and cook in the pot for 10 minutes, stirring frequently; set aside. Add the leek, garlic, carrots, and celery to the pot and cook for 4 minutes. Put the beef back to the pot among pearl barley, bay leaf, beef broth, and soy sauce. Seal the lid, select Manual, and cook for 30 minutes on High pressure. When done, allow a natural release for 10 minutes, then perform a quick pressure release and unlock the lid. Discard the bay leaf. Adjust the taste and top with Parmesan cheese. Serve right away.

Mushroom Chicken Soup

INGREDIENTS for Servings: 4

1 tbsp. olive oil	4 cups low-sodium chicken stock
7 oz. chicken breast	
1 onion, finely chopped	Salt and pepper, to taste
2 cups sliced button mushrooms	¼ cup heavy whipping cream

DIRECTIONS and Cooking Time: 20 Minutes
Press the Sauté bottom on the Electric Pressure Cooker. Add and heat the olive oil. Add the chicken breast and sauté for 3 to 4 minutes to evenly brown. Add the onions and sauté for 3 minutes or until translucent and softened. Add the mushrooms and stock. Sprinkle with salt and pepper. Lock the lid. Press the Manual bottom in the pot. Set the timer to 15 minutes at High Pressure. Once the timer goes off, press Cancel. Do a quick pressure release. Open the lid, mix in the cream, transfer them in a large bowl and serve.

Kale And Veal Stew

INGREDIENTS for Servings: 6

1 tbsp. olive oil	10 oz. fat removed and chopped veal shoulder
2 large onions, finely chopped	
1 small sweet potato, diced	1 lb. fresh kale, chopped
4 cups low-sodium beef stock	Salt and pepper, to taste

DIRECTIONS and Cooking Time: 35 Minutes
Press the Sauté bottom on the Electric Pressure Cooker. Add and heat the olive oil. Add the onions and sauté for 3 minutes until turn translucent and softened. Add the sweet potato and ¼ cup of stock. Sauté for 5 minutes or until soft. Add the remaining stock, veal shoulder, and kale to the Electric Pressure Cooker. Sprinkle with salt and pepper. Combine to mix well. Lock the lid. Press Manual. Set the timer to 25 minutes at High pressure. Once the timer goes off, press Cancel. Do a quick pressure release. Open the lid, transfer them in a large bowl and serve

Easy Veggie Soup

INGREDIENTS for Servings: 4

1 cup okra, trimmed	2 cups Vegetable broth
1 Carrot, sliced	
1 cup Broccoli florets	1 tbsp Lemon juice
1 green Bell Pepper,	4 Garlic cloves,

sliced 1 red Bell Pepper, sliced 1 Onion, sliced	minced Salt and black pepper to taste 1 tbsp Olive oil

DIRECTIONS and Cooking Time: 40 Minutes
Warm olive oil in your Electric Pressure Cooker on Sauté. Place the onion and garlic and cook for 1 minute. Add in carrot, okra, broccoli florets, green bell pepper, and red bell pepper and cook for 5-10 minutes. Stir in vegetable broth, salt, and black pepper and seal the lid. Select Meat/Stew and cook for 15 minutes on High pressure. When done, perform a quick pressure release and unlock the lid. Sprinkle with lemon juice and divide between bowls before serving.

Seafood And Vegetable Ragout

INGREDIENTS for Servings: 4

2 tablespoons olive oil 1 shallot, diced 2 carrots, diced 1 parsnip, diced 1 teaspoon fresh garlic, minced 1/2 cup dry white wine 2 cups fish stock 1 tomato, pureed	1 bay leaf 1 pound shrimp, deveined 1/2 pound scallops Seasoned salt and freshly ground pepper, to taste 1 tablespoon paprika 2 tablespoons fresh parsley, chopped 1 lime, sliced

DIRECTIONS and Cooking Time: 20 Minutes
Press the "Sauté" button and heat the oil. Now, sauté the shallot, carrot, and parsnip for 4 to 5 minutes or until they are tender. Stir in the garlic and continue to sauté an additional 30 second or until aromatic. Stir in the white wine, stock, tomato, bay leaf, shrimp, scallops, salt, black pepper, and paprika. Secure the lid. Choose the "Manual" mode. Cook for 5 minutes at High pressure. Once cooking is complete, use a natural pressure release for 5 minutes; carefully remove the lid. Serve garnished with fresh parsley and lime slices. Enjoy!

Kale, Potato & Beef Stew

INGREDIENTS for Servings: 2

1 green bell pepper, chopped 2 medium potatoes, chopped ½ pound beef stew meat, cut into cubes 1 small onion, chopped 1 celery stalk, chopped	1 tbsp hot sauce 1 tbsp olive oil ½ tsp garlic powder 2 carrots, peeled and chopped 1 cup kale, trimmed and chopped 2 cups beef broth Salt and black pepper to taste

DIRECTIONS and Cooking Time: 55 Minutes
Warm olive oil in your Electric Pressure Cooker on Sauté Place the meat and cook for 4-5 minutes until browned. Stir in potatoes, hot sauce, onion, celery, garlic powder, bell pepper, carrots, kale leaves, beef broth, salt, and black pepper. Seal the lid, select Meat/Stew, and cook for 40 minutes. When done, perform a quick pressure release. Serve warm.

Electric Pressure Cooker Ham And Potato Soup

INGREDIENTS for Servings: 5

2 tablespoons butter 1 onion, diced 8 cloves of garlic, minced 2 pounds Yukon Gold potatoes, cut into small chunks A dash of cayenne pepper	4 cups chicken broth ½ cup cheddar cheese, grated 1 cup cooked ham, diced Salt and pepper 2 tablespoons fried bacon bits

DIRECTIONS and Cooking Time: 30 Minutes
Press the Sauté button on the Electric Pressure Cooker. Heat the butter and sauté the onions and garlic until fragrant.3. Stir in the potatoes and cook for 3 minutes. Pour in the broth, cayenne pepper, cheese, and cooked ham. Season with salt and pepper to taste. Close the lid and press the Manual button. Adjust the cooking time to 25 minutes. Do quick pressure release. Open the lid and garnish with bacon bits on top.

Mom's Pork Vegetable Soup

INGREDIENTS for Servings: 4

1 pound pork stew meat, cubed 2 cups spinach Sea salt and ground black pepper, to taste 1 celery, sliced 1 carrot, sliced	1 turnip, peeled and sliced 4 cups beef bone broth 1 cup scallion, chopped 1 tablespoon olive oil

DIRECTIONS and Cooking Time: 40 Minutes
Press the "Sauté" button to preheat your Electric Pressure Cooker; heat the oil. Now, sear the meat until it is delicately browned. Add the remaining ingredients, except for the spinach. Secure the lid. Choose the "Soup" setting and cook at High pressure for 30 minutes. Once cooking is complete, use a quick pressure release; carefully remove the lid. Add the spinach to the Electric Pressure Cooker; seal the lid and allow it to sit in the residual heat until wilted. Ladle the soup into individual bowls and serve right away. Bon appétit!

Coconut Seafood Soup

INGREDIENTS for Servings: 5

1 cup coconut milk 10 shrimps, shelled and deveined 1 thumb-size ginger, crushed	4 tilapia fillets 2 cups water Salt and pepper, to taste

DIRECTIONS and Cooking Time: 8 Minutes
Place all ingredients in the Electric Pressure Cooker. Stir to combine well. Lock the lid. Set on the Manual mode, then set the timer to 8 minutes at Low Pressure. When the timer goes off, perform a quick release. Carefully open the lid. Allow to cool before serving.

Chicken, Shrimp And Sausage Gumbo

INGREDIENTS for Servings: 4

2 tablespoons olive oil 1 onion, diced 1 teaspoon garlic, minced 1/2 pound chicken breasts, boneless, skinless and cubed 1/2 pound smoked chicken sausage, cut into slices 2 sweet peppers, diced 1 jalapeno pepper, minced 1 celery stalk, diced 2 cups chicken bone broth 2 tomatoes, chopped	1 tablespoon Creole seasoning Sea salt and ground black pepper, to taste 1 teaspoon cayenne pepper 1 tablespoon oyster sauce 1 bay leaf 1 pound shrimp, deveined 1/2 pound okra, frozen 2 stalks green onions, sliced thinly 1 tablespoon fresh lemon juice

DIRECTIONS and Cooking Time: 25 Minutes
Press the "Sauté" button and heat the oil. Sweat the onion and garlic until tender and aromatic or about 3 minutes; reserve. Then, heat the remaining tablespoon of olive oil and cook the chicken and sausage until no longer pink, about 4 minutes. Make sure to stir periodically to ensure even cooking. Stir in the peppers, celery, broth, tomatoes, Creole seasoning, salt, black pepper, cayenne pepper, oyster sauce, and bay leaf. Add the reserved onion mixture. Secure the lid. Choose the "Manual" mode. Cook for 7 minutes at High pressure. Once cooking is complete, use a quick pressure release; carefully remove the lid. Afterwards, stir in the shrimp and okra. Secure the lid. Choose the "Manual" mode. Cook for 3 minutes at High pressure. Once cooking is complete, use a natural pressure release; carefully remove the lid. Divide between individual bowls and garnish with green onions. Drizzle lemon juice over each serving. Bon appétit!

Chicken Soup With Vegetables

INGREDIENTS for Servings: 4

1 beet, chopped 1 carrot, diced ½ pound.chicken breasts, cooked, shredded ½ celery, diced 1 onion, chopped 1 cup mushrooms, sliced	5 cups chicken stock 2 garlic cloves, chopped 1 tsp thyme 1 tsp rosemary 2 bay leaves 2 tbsp olive oil Salt and black pepper to taste

DIRECTIONS and Cooking Time: 35 Minutes
Warm olive oil in your Electric Pressure Cooker on Sauté. Place the carrots, beet, and onion and cook for 2-3 minutes. Add in garlic, celery, and mushrooms and cook for 3 more minutes. Put in chicken breasts, chicken stock, thyme, rosemary, bay leaves, salt, and black pepper. Seal the lid, select Soup, and cook on Low pressure. When done, perform a quick pressure release and unlock the lid. Serve warm.

Seafood Chowder With Bacon And Celery

INGREDIENTS for Servings: 4

3 strips bacon, chopped 1 onion, chopped 2 stalks celery, diced 2 cloves garlic, minced 1 tablespoon Creole seasoning Sea salt and ground black pepper, to taste	2 carrots, diced 3 cups seafood stock 2 ripe tomatoes, pureed 2 tablespoons tomato paste 2 bay leaves 1 pound clams, chopped 1 ½ tablespoons flaxseed meal

DIRECTIONS and Cooking Time: 15 Minutes
Press the "Sauté" button to preheat your Electric Pressure Cooker. Now, cook the bacon until it is crisp; crumble the bacon and set it aside. Now, sauté the onion, carrot, celery, and garlic in bacon drippings. Add the remaining ingredients, except for the chopped clams, to the inner pot. Secure the lid. Choose the "Manual" mode and cook for 4 minutes at High pressure. Once cooking is complete, use a quick pressure release; carefully remove the lid. Stir in the chopped clams and flaxseed meal. Press the "Sauté" button and let it simmer for 2 to 3 minutes longer or until everything is heated through. Serve in individual bowls topped with the reserved bacon. Bon appétit!

Hearty Irish Burgoo

INGREDIENTS for Servings: 8

2 bell peppers, chopped	Sea salt and ground black pepper, to taste
2 chicken thighs, boneless	2 carrots, chopped
2 pounds pork butt roast, cut into 2-inch pieces	4 garlic cloves, chopped
3 tablespoons Worcestershire sauce	4 cups beef bone broth
1 cup beer	1 pound frozen corn kernels
1 (28-ounce) can tomatoes, crushed	1 tablespoon lard, melted
2 pounds beef stew meat, cut into 2-inch pieces	1 red chili pepper, chopped
	1 onion, chopped

DIRECTIONS and Cooking Time: 30 Minutes
Press the "Sauté" button and melt the lard. Once hot, brown the meat in batches. Remove the browned meats to a bowl. Then, sauté the peppers, onion, carrots for about 3 minutes or until tender and fragrant. Add the garlic and continue to cook for 30 seconds more. Add the meat back to the Electric Pressure Cooker. Stir in the remaining ingredients, except for the corn kernels. Secure the lid. Choose the "Meat/Stew" mode and cook for 20 minutes at High pressure. Once cooking is complete, use a quick pressure release; carefully remove the lid. Lastly, stir in the corn and continue to cook for a few minutes more on the "Sauté" function. Serve immediately.

Beef Borscht Soup

INGREDIENTS for Servings: 6

3 beets, peeled and diced	2 pounds ground beef
3 stalks of celery, diced	1 onion, diced
2 large carrots, diced	3 cups shredded cabbage
2 cloves of garlic, diced	6 cups beef stock
	1 bay leaf
	½ tablespoon thyme
	Salt and pepper

DIRECTIONS and Cooking Time: 20 Minutes
Press the Sauté button on the Electric Pressure Cooker. Sauté the beef for 5 minutes until slightly golden. Add all the rest of the ingredients in the Electric Pressure Cooker. Close the lid and press the Manual button. Adjust the cooking time to 15 minutes. Do natural pressure release.

Three Beans Mix Chili

INGREDIENTS for Servings: 4

1 tablespoon olive oil	¼ dried kidney beans, rinsed, soaked for 8 hours and drained
1 cup onion, chopped	
½ green bell pepper, seeded and chopped	1 cup fresh tomatoes, chopped
½ cup carrot, peeled and chopped	1 cup homemade tomato paste
2 tablespoons celery stalk, chopped	1 teaspoon dried oregano, crushed
½ tablespoon garlic, minced	1 tablespoon mild chili powder
¼ cup dried pinto beans, rinsed, soaked for 8 hours and drained	½ teaspoon smoked paprika
	½ teaspoons ground cumin
¼ cup dried black beans, rinsed, soaked for 8 hours and drained	¼ teaspoon ground coriander
	2 cups low-sodium vegetable broth

DIRECTIONS and Cooking Time: 20 Minutes
Select the 'sauté' function on the Electric Pressure Cooker, add the oil, bell pepper, celery, onion, carrot and garlic, and cook for 5 minutes. Add the remaining ingredients to the pot then secure the lid. Select the 'manual' function and set to high pressure. Cook for 15 minutes. After the beep, use the 'natural release' function to vent the steam, then remove the lid. Garnish with scallion* and serve.

Butternut Squash Curry Soup

INGREDIENTS for Servings: 4

1 tsp olive oil	1 butternut squash, peeled and cut into 1-inch cubes
1 large onion, chopped	
2 cloves garlic, minced	1½ tsp salt
3 cups water	1 tbsp curry powder
	½ cup coconut milk

DIRECTIONS and Cooking Time: 50 Minutes
Preheat the Electric Pressure Cooker by selecting SAUTÉ. Add and heat the oil. Add the onion and sauté for about 5 minutes, until softened. Add the garlic and cook for another 1 minute. Press the CANCEL key to stop the SAUTÉ function. Pour in the water and add the squash. Sprinkle with salt and curry powder and stir well. Select the SOUP setting and set the cooking time for 30 minutes. When the timer beeps, use a quick release. Carefully unlock the lid. With an immersion blender, blend the soup until smooth. Pour in the coconut milk and mix well. Serve with dried cranberries and pumpkin seeds.

Japanese-style Tofu Soup

INGREDIENTS for Servings: 4

½ cup corn 2 tbsp miso paste 1 onion, sliced 1 cup silken tofu, cubed 2 celery stalks, chopped	1 tsp wakame flakes 2 carrots, chopped Salt and black pepper to taste Soy sauce, to taste 2 tsp dashi granules

DIRECTIONS and Cooking Time: 15 Minutes
Add all ingredients, except miso paste and soy sauce. Pour in 4 cups of water. Seal the lid, select Manual, and cook for 7 minutes at High. Do a quick pressure release. Mix miso paste with 1 cup of broth. Stir it into soup. Add soy sauce and stir. Serve.

Veggie Cheese Soup
INGREDIENTS for Servings: 4-6

1 package vegetables, frozen 1 can cream mushroom soup 1 jar cheese sauce	Salt and ground black pepper to taste Mozzarella cheese, shredded

DIRECTIONS and Cooking Time: 30 Minutes
Add the vegetables to the Electric Pressure Cooker. Pour in the mushroom soup and cheese sauce, stir well. Sprinkle with salt and pepper, stir. Top with Mozzarella cheese. Close and lock the lid. Select MANUAL and cook at HIGH pressure for 7 minutes. Once timer goes off, allow to Naturally Release for 10 minutes, then release any remaining pressure manually. Uncover the pot. Serve.

Cheddar Cheese And Broccoli Soup
INGREDIENTS for Servings: 4

2 cups vegetable broth ½ cup onions, chopped ½ cup parsnip, chopped 1 cup carrots, sliced Salt and black pepper to taste	1 cup bell peppers, chopped 1 cup fennel bulb, sliced 2 cups broccoli florets ½ cup cheddar cheese, grated

DIRECTIONS and Cooking Time: 15 Minutes
Place all ingredients, except for the cheddar cheese, in your IP and seal the lid. Select Manual and cook for 3 minutes at High. Do a quick pressure release. Puree soup with a hand blender. Serve soup topped with freshly grated cheddar cheese.

Vegetable Mediterranean Delight Stew
INGREDIENTS for Servings: 5

1 butternut squash, cubed ½ tsp ground turmeric ½ tsp ground cumin 1 clove garlic, minced 1/3 cup raisins 1 cup vegetable broth 1 carrot, sliced thin 1 ripe tomato, chopped 1 (8-oz) can tomato sauce	1 cup onion, chopped 1 (10-oz) package frozen okra, thawed 2 cups zucchini, cubed 2 cups eggplants, sliced ¼ tsp crushed red pepper ¼ tsp ground cinnamon ¼ tsp paprika Goat cheese for garnish

DIRECTIONS and Cooking Time: 38 Minutes
Stir all the ingredients, except for goat cheese, in your IP, and stir to combine. Seal the lid, select Manual at High, and cook for 8 minutes. When ready, release the pressure naturally for 5 minutes. Top with goat cheese.

Easy Vegetarian Ratatouille
INGREDIENTS for Servings: 4

1 pound eggplant, cut into rounds 1 tablespoon sea salt 3 tablespoons olive oil 1 red onion, sliced 4 cloves garlic, minced 4 sweet peppers, seeded and chopped 1 red chili pepper, seeded and minced	Sea salt and ground black pepper, to taste 1 teaspoon capers 1/2 teaspoon celery seeds 2 tomatoes, pureed 1 cup roasted vegetable broth 2 tablespoons coriander, chopped

DIRECTIONS and Cooking Time: 25 Minutes
Toss the eggplant with 1 tablespoon of sea salt; allow it to drain in a colander. Press the "Sauté" button and heat the olive oil. Sauté the onion until tender and translucent, about 4 minutes. Add the garlic and continue to sauté for 30 seconds more or until fragrant. Add the remaining ingredients to the inner pot, including the drained eggplant. Secure the lid. Choose the "Manual" mode. Cook for 7 minutes at High pressure. Once cooking is complete, use a quick pressure release; carefully remove the lid. Press the "Sauté" button and cook on low setting until the ratatouille has thickened or about 7 minutes. Bon appétit!

Chicken & Noodle Soup
INGREDIENTS for Servings: 2

8 oz egg noodles 2 Carrots, sliced 1 tbsp Olive Oil 1 small onion,	1 garlic clove, minced Salt and black pepper to taste 1 small Bay Leaf

chopped 2 Celery Ribs, diced 1 small Banana Pepper, minced	2 Chicken Breasts, skinless 3 cups Chicken Broth

DIRECTIONS and Cooking Time: 40 Minutes
Warm olive oil in your Electric Pressure Cooker on Sauté. Place the onion, celery, carrots, garlic, banana pepper, salt, and black pepper and cook for 4 minutes. Add in bay leaf, chicken breast, and chicken broth. Seal the lid, select Manual, and cook for 15 minutes on High pressure. When done, perform a quick pressure release and unlock the lid. Transfer the chicken onto a cutting board and shred it. Put the chicken back to the pot among egg noodles and cook for 7-8 minutes on Sauté. Divide between bowls and serve.

Potato And Corn Soup
INGREDIENTS for Servings: 4

1 cup fresh corn kernels 1 tablespoon unsalted butter, melted ½ medium onion, chopped 1 celery stalk, chopped 1 garlic clove, chopped1 large russet potato, peeled and chopped	1 ½ carrots, peeled and chopped 1 tablespoon dried parsley, crushed 3 cups vegetable broth 1½ tablespoon corn starch Freshly ground black pepper, to taste ¼ cup water

DIRECTIONS and Cooking Time: 12 Minutes
Pour the melted butter into the Electric Pressure Cooker and press the 'sauté' key. Add the celery, onion, carrot and garlic to the pot, then cook for 3 minutes. Now add the broth, potatoes, corns, black pepper and parsley to the pot, and secure the lid. Select the 'manual' function, set to high pressure and the timer to 6 minutes. After the beep, 'quick release' the steam and remove the lid. Meanwhile, prepare the corn starch slurry by mixing it with some water. Pour the corn starch slurry into the soup, stirring continuously. Set the cooker to the 'sauté' function and cook for 3 minutes. Serve hot

Chinese-style Chicken Stew With Broccoli
INGREDIENTS for Servings: 4 上

1 tsp Chinese Five Spice seasoning 1 cup Coconut Aminos 4 Chicken Breasts 1 cup Chicken Broth 3 tbsp Olive oil	1 inch Ginger, grated Salt and black pepper to taste 4 cups Broccoli Florets 1 tbsp Sesame seeds

½ tsp Fish Sauce 1 garlic clove, minced	2 tbsp Arrowroot Flour 2 tbsp Water

DIRECTIONS and Cooking Time: 25 Minutes
Place the chicken breasts, chicken broth, olive oil, garlic, ginger, coconut aminos, Chinese five spice seasoning, black pepper, and salt in your Electric Pressure Cooker. Seal the lid, select Manual, and cook for 8 minutes on High pressure. When done, perform a quick pressure release. Whisk the arrowroot with water in a bowl and pour it into the pot. Add in broccoli and cook for 5 minutes on Sauté. Stir in plain vinegar. Serve garnished with sesame seeds.

Beef And Cabbage Soup
INGREDIENTS for Servings: 4-6

2 tbsp coconut oil 1 onion, diced 1 clove garlic, minced 14 oz can diced tomatoes, undrained	1 lb ground beef 4 cups water Salt and ground black pepper to taste 1 head cabbage, chopped

DIRECTIONS and Cooking Time: 35 Minutes
Preheat the Electric Pressure Cooker by selecting SAUTÉ. Add and heat the oil. Add the onion and garlic and sauté for 2 minutes. Add the beef and cook, stirring, for 2-3 minutes until lightly brown. Pour in the water and tomatoes. Season with salt and pepper, stir well. Press the CANCEL key to stop the SAUTÉ function. Close and lock the lid. Select MANUAL and cook at HIGH pressure for 12 minutes. When the timer goes off, use a Quick Release. Carefully open the lid. Add the cabbage, select SAUTÉ and simmer for 5 minutes. Serve.

Butternut Squash & Apple Soup
INGREDIENTS for Servings: 6

3 lb butternut squash, chopped 3 tbsp butter ¾ cup cranberries 1 tbsp cinnamon	4 apples, chopped ½ white onion, chopped Salt and black pepper to taste

DIRECTIONS and Cooking Time: 29 Minutes
Melt butter on Sauté and cook onion for 3 minutes. Pour in the remaining ingredients and 6 cups of water, except for the cranberries. Seal the lid, select Manual at High, and cook for 6 minutes. When done, release the pressure quickly. Puree the soup with an immersion blender until smooth. Serve topped with cranberries.

Meatball Soup

INGREDIENTS for Servings: 4-6

1 tbsp olive oil	1 can diced tomatoes
1 onion, chopped	1 green bell pepper, chopped
2 cloves garlic, minced	½ tsp cumin
1 package prepared meatballs	1 tbsp oregano
1 cup carrots, chopped finely	Salt and ground black pepper to taste
	1 egg, beaten

DIRECTIONS and Cooking Time: 35 Minutes
Select the SAUTÉ setting on the Electric Pressure Cooker and heat the oil. Add the onion and garlic, sauté for 1-2 minutes, or until fragrant. Add the meatballs and cook for 4-5 minutes, until the meat has browned all over. Add the carrot, tomatoes, bell pepper, cumin, oregano, salt and black pepper, stir well. Close and lock the lid. Press the CANCEL button to stop the SAUTE function, then select the SOUP setting and set the cooking time for 15 minutes at HIGH pressure. When the timer beeps, use a Quick Release. Carefully unlock the lid. Return to SAUTÉ. Add the beaten egg. And cook for 3-4 minutes. Serve.

Vegetarian Minestrone With Navy Beans

INGREDIENTS for Servings: 2-4

2 tbsp olive oil	¼ tsp black pepper
1 onion, diced	2 bay leaves
1 cup celery, chopped	28 ounces canned diced tomatoes
1 carrot, peeled and diced	6 ounces canned tomato paste
1 green bell pepper, chopped	2 cups kale
2 cloves garlic, minced	14 oz canned Navy beans, rinsed, drained
3 cups chicken broth	½ cup white rice
½ tsp dried parsley	¼ cup Parmesan cheese, shredded
½ tsp dried thyme	
½ tsp dried oregano	
½ tsp salt	

DIRECTIONS and Cooking Time: 25 Minutes
Warm olive oil on Sauté. Stir in carrot, celery and onion and cook for 5 to 6 minutes until soft. Add garlic and bell pepper and cook for 2 minutes as you stir until aromatic. Stir in pepper, thyme, stock, salt, parsley, oregano, tomatoes, bay leaves, and tomato paste to dissolve. Mix in rice. Seal the lid and cook on High Pressure for 15 minutes. Do a quick release. Add kale to the liquid and stir. Use residual heat in slightly wilting the greens. Discard bay leaves. Stir in navy beans and serve topped with Parmesan cheese.

Lentil & Bell Pepper Soup

INGREDIENTS for Servings: 2-4

1 cup red lentils, soaked overnight	½ tsp ground black pepper
1 red bell pepper, seeded and chopped	½ tsp cumin, ground
	½ tsp salt
1 onion, peeled, chopped	2 tbsp olive oil
½ cup carrot puree	A handful of parsley, to garnish

DIRECTIONS and Cooking Time: 35 Minutes
Heat the oil on Sauté, add stir-fry the onions for 4 minutes. Add the remaining ingredients and pour in 4 cups of water. Seal the lid and cook on Soup/Broth mode for 30 minutes on High Pressure. Do a quick Pressure release. Sprinkle with fresh parsley and serve warm.

Corn And Potato Chowder

INGREDIENTS for Servings: 4

1 sweet onion, chopped	2 tablespoons butter
2 garlic cloves, minced	1 pound potatoes, cut into bite-sized pieces
1 sweet pepper, deveined and sliced	3 cups creamed corn kernels
1 jalapeno pepper, deveined and sliced	1 cup double cream
4 tablespoons all-purpose flour	Kosher salt and ground black pepper, to taste
4 cups vegetable broth	1/2 teaspoon cayenne pepper

DIRECTIONS and Cooking Time: 25 Minutes
Press the "Sauté" button and melt the butter. Once hot, sauté the sweet onions, garlic, and peppers for about 3 minutes or until they are tender and fragrant. Sprinkle the flour over the vegetables; continue stirring approximately 4 minutes or until your vegetables are coated. Add the broth and potatoes and gently stir to combine. Secure the lid. Choose the "Manual" mode and cook for 5 minutes at High pressure. Once cooking is complete, use a quick pressure release; carefully remove the lid. Press the "Sauté" button and use the lowest setting. Stir in the creamed corn, double cream, salt, black pepper, and cayenne pepper. Let it simmer, stirring continuously for about 5 minutes or until everything is thoroughly heated. Taste and adjust the seasonings. Bon appétit!

Minestrone Soup

INGREDIENTS for Servings: 4

2 tablespoons olive oil	1 28 oz.) can San Marzano tomatoes
2 stalks celery, diced	
1 large onion, diced	1 15 oz.) can white or

1 large carrot, diced 3 cloves garlic, minced 1 teaspoon dried oregano 1 teaspoon dried basil Sea salt and pepper to taste	cannellini beans 4 cups bone broth or vegetable broth 1 bay leaf ½ cup fresh spinach 1 cup gluten-free elbow pasta 1/3 cup finely grated parmesan cheese 2 tablespoons fresh pesto

DIRECTIONS and Cooking Time: 6 Minutes
Switch the Electric Pressure Cooker to 'sauté' mode and add the oil, onion, garlic, celery and carrot. Cook for 3 minutes. Drizzle the salt, pepper, oregano and basil into the mix to add more flavour. Add the broth, spinach, pasta, tomatoes and bay leaf to the pot and select 'manual' settings. Cook for 6 minutes at high pressure. Let it sit for 2 minutes after the beep, then 'quick release' the steam. Remove the lid carefully. Stir in the white beans. Serve with a grating of parmesan cheese and pesto on top.

Leek Soup With Tofu
INGREDIENTS for Servings: 2-4

3 large leeks 3 tbsp butter 1 onion, chopped 1 lb potatoes, chopped 5 cups vegetable stock 2 tsp lemon juice	¼ tsp nutmeg ¼ tsp ground coriander 1 bay leaf 5 oz silken tofu Salt and white pepper Freshly snipped chives, to garnish

DIRECTIONS and Cooking Time: 25 Minutes
Remove most of the green parts of the leeks. Slice the white parts very finely. Melt butter on Sauté, and stir-fry leeks and onion for 5 minutes without browning. Add potatoes, stock, juice, nutmeg, coriander and bay leaf. Season to taste with salt and pepper, and seal the lid. Press Manual/Pressure Cook and set the timer to 10 minutes. Cook on High Pressure. Do a quick release and discard the bay leaf. Process the soup in a food processor until smooth. Season to taste, add silken tofu. Serve the soup sprinkled with freshly snipped chives.

VEGETABLE & VEGETARIAN RECIPES

Onion & Chickpea Stew

INGREDIENTS for Servings: 2-4

1 cup chickpeas, soaked	3 cups vegetable broth
3 purple onions, peeled and chopped	1 tbsp paprika
2 tomatoes, roughly chopped	3 tbsp butter
2 oz fresh parsley, chopped	2 tbsp olive oil
	1 tsp salt
	½ tsp black pepper

DIRECTIONS and Cooking Time: 35 Minutes
Warm oil on Sauté and stir-fry the onions for 3 minutes. Add the rest of the ingredients. Seal the lid and cook on the Meat/Stew for 30 minutes on High. Do a quick release and serve warm.

Steamed Vegetables

INGREDIENTS for Servings: 2-4

3 small zucchinis, sliced (1 inch thick)	1 cup water
2 bell peppers, sliced (1 inch thick)	1 tbsp Italian herb mix
½ cup garlic, peeled and minced	Salt to taste
	2 tbsp olive oil

DIRECTIONS and Cooking Time: 15 Minutes
Prepare the Electric Pressure Cooker by adding the water to the pot and placing the steam rack in it. In a large bowl, combine the zucchinis, peppers, and garlic. Season the veggies with Italian herb mix, salt and oil. Stir well. Place the vegetables on the rack. Close and lock the lid. Select the STEAM setting and set the cooking time for 7 minutes. When the timer beeps, use a Quick Release. Carefully unlock the lid. Serve.

Cheesy Potatoes With Herbs

INGREDIENTS for Servings: 4

2 tbsp butter	½ tsp basil
1 lb potatoes, cubed	½ tsp cayenne pepper
1 cup chicken broth	Salt to taste
½ tsp rosemary	½ cup Romano cheese, shredded
½ tsp thyme	

DIRECTIONS and Cooking Time: 25 Minutes
Melt the butter in your Electric Pressure Cooker on Sauté. Place the potatoes and cook for 5 minutes. Add in chicken broth, rosemary, thyme, and basil and seal the lid. Select Manual and cook for 5 minutes on High pressure. Once over, allow a natural release for 10 minutes and unlock the lid. Sprinkle with salt and cayenne pepper and transfer to a plate. Scatter Romano cheese over and serve.

Easy Vegan Posole

INGREDIENTS for Servings: 4

2 dried pasilla chili peppers, seeded and minced	1/2 pound dried hominy, soaked overnight and rinsed
1 teaspoon cumin seeds	4 cups water
1 teaspoon garlic, sliced	2 Roma tomatoes, chopped
Kosher salt and ground black pepper, to taste	1 tablespoon bouillon granules
1 onion, chopped	2 bay leaves
	1 cup radishes, sliced

DIRECTIONS and Cooking Time: 1 Hour
Put the chilis in a bowl with hot water; let them soak for 15 minutes until soft. Transfer the chilis to your food processor; add the cumin seeds, garlic, salt, and black pepper. Add 1 cup of water to the food processor and puree the mixture until well blended. Transfer the mixture to your Electric Pressure Cooker. Add the onion, hominy, water, tomatoes, bouillon granules, and bay leaves to the inner pot. Secure the lid. Choose the "Soup/Broth" mode and cook for 40 minutes at High pressure. Once cooking is complete, use a quick pressure release; carefully remove the lid. Serve warm, garnished with fresh radishes. Bon appétit!

Sautéed Spinach & Leeks With Blue Cheese

INGREDIENTS for Servings: 2

9 oz fresh spinach	½ cup blue cheese, crumbled
2 leeks, chopped	3 tbsp olive oil
2 red onions, chopped	1 tbsp salt
2 garlic cloves, crushed	

DIRECTIONS and Cooking Time: 10 Minutes
Grease the inner pot with oil. Stir-fry leeks, garlic, and onions, for about 5 minutes, on Sauté mode. Add spinach and give it a good stir. Season with salt and cook for 3 more minutes, stirring constantly. Press Cancel, Transfer to a serving dish and sprinkle with blue cheese. Serve right away.

Vegetable One-pot

INGREDIENTS for Servings: 4

1 zucchini, sliced	¼ cup fresh parsley, chopped
2 tbsp olive oil	1 cup water
1 tsp salt	2 carrots, chopped
2 tomatoes, chopped	1 tsp garlic, minced
½ lb green beans	1 onion, chopped

| ½ lb sweet potatoes, cubed | |

DIRECTIONS and Cooking Time: 35 Minutes
Set your IP to Sauté and heat olive oil. Add onion, zucchini, carrots, garlic, salt, and pepper, and cook for 5 minutes. Add in the remaining ingredients, except for the parsley. Seal the lid, select Manual at High, and cook for 12 minutes. When done, release the pressure naturally for 5 minutes. Serve sprinkled with parsley.

Zucchini And Bell Pepper Stir Fry

INGREDIENTS for Servings: 6

2 large zucchinis, sliced	1 tbsp. coconut oil
4 garlic cloves, minced	1 onion, chopped
2 red sweet bell peppers, julienned	Salt and pepper, to taste
	¼ cup water

DIRECTIONS and Cooking Time: 5 Minutes
Press the Sauté button on the Electric Pressure Cooker. Heat the coconut oil and sauté the onion and garlic for 2 minutes or until fragrant. Add the zucchini and red bell peppers. Sprinkle salt and pepper for seasoning. Pour in the water. Lock the lid. Set the Electric Pressure Cooker to Manual mode, then set the timer for 5 minutes at High Pressure. Once cooking is complete, do a quick pressure release. Carefully open the lid. Serve warm.

Spicy Pickled Potatoes

INGREDIENTS for Servings: 4

1 tablespoon cumin seeds	1 teaspoon salt
1 tablespoon coriander seeds, pounded	1 teaspoon dry pomegranate powder
5 cloves	2 teaspoons dried fenugreek leaves
1 bay leaf	1 tablespoon mango pickle
½ teaspoon red chili powder	2 tablespoon oil
½ teaspoon turmeric powder	5 potatoes, boiled and cubed

DIRECTIONS and Cooking Time: 4 Minutes
Add the oil and all the spices in the Electric Pressure Cooker and 'sauté' for 1 minute. Add the remaining ingredients to the pot and secure the lid. Use the 'manual' function on your Electric Pressure Cooker to cook for 3 minutes at high pressure. After the beep, 'Quick release' the steam and remove the lid. Stir well to coat the potatoes and serve hot.

Mixed Vegetables Medley

INGREDIENTS for Servings: 4

1 small head broccoli, broken into florets	16 asparagus, trimmed
1 small head cauliflower, broken into florets	5 ounces green beans
	2 carrots, peeled and cut on bias
	Salt to taste

DIRECTIONS and Cooking Time: 15 Minutes
Add 1 cup of water and set trivet on top of water and place steamer basket on top. In an even layer, spread green beans, broccoli, cauliflower, asparagus, and carrots in the steamer basket. Seal the lid and cook on Steam for 3 minutes on High. Release the pressure quickly. Remove basket from the pot and season with salt.

Electric Pressure Cooker French Onion Soup

INGREDIENTS for Servings: 4

6 tablespoon unsalted butter	1 teaspoon apple cider vinegar
3 pounds onions, chopped	½ cup dry sherry
Salt and pepper to taste	1 pound cheese, grated
3 cups chicken stock	1 tablespoon chives for garnish
1 bay leaf	8 slices of bread, toasted
2 sprigs of thyme	
1 teaspoon fish sauce	

DIRECTIONS and Cooking Time: 2 Minutes
Press the Sauté button on the Electric Pressure Cooker. Heat the butter and sauté the onion for 10 minutes until caramelized. Stir constantly. Season with salt and pepper and stir in the rest of the ingredients except for the bread. Stir to combine everything. Place the slices of bread on top. Close the lid and press the Manual button. Adjust the cooking time to 10 minutes. Do natural pressure release.

Maple-glazed Acorn Squash

INGREDIENTS for Servings: 2-4

½ cup water	2 tbsp butter
3 tablespoons maple syrup	1 tbsp dark brown sugar
1 lb acorn squash, cut into 2-inch chunks	1 tbsp cinnamon
	Salt and ground black pepper to taste

DIRECTIONS and Cooking Time: 30 Minutes
In a small bowl, mix 1 tablespoon maple syrup and water. Pour into the pot. Add in squash, seal the lid and cook on High Pressure for 4 minutes. Release the pressure quickly. Transfer the squash to a serving dish. Set on Sauté. Mix sugar, cinnamon, the remaining 2 tbsp maple syrup and the liquid in the pot. Cook as you stir for 4 minutes to obtain a thick consistency and starts to turn caramelized and golden. Spread honey glaze over squash; add pepper and salt to taste.

Pumpkin & Potato Mash

INGREDIENTS for Servings: 4

½ lb pumpkin, cubed	½ cup milk
½ lb sweet potatoes, cubed	2 tbsp butter
2 garlic cloves	½ cup Parmesan cheese, grated
¼ tsp dried tarragon	Salt and black pepper to taste
¼ tsp dried sage	

DIRECTIONS and Cooking Time: 20 Minutes
Pour 1 cup of water in your Electric Pressure Cooker and fit in a steamer basket. Place the pumpkin, sweet potatoes, and garlic in the steamer basket and seal the lid. Select Manual and cook for 12 minutes on High pressure. Once ready, perform a quick pressure release and unlock the lid. Remove the veggies to a bowl. Stir in tarragon and sage. Pour in milk and butter and them using a potato masher until smooth; adjust the seasonings. Sprinkle with Parmesan cheese and serve.

Tomato, Lentil & Quinoa Stew

INGREDIENTS for Servings: 2-4

1 cup quinoa, soaked overnight	1 cup tomatoes, diced
1 cup lentils, soaked overnight	1 tsp garlic, minced
	4 cups beef broth
¼ cup sun-dried tomatoes, chopped	1 tsp salt
	1 tsp red pepper flakes

DIRECTIONS and Cooking Time: 25 Minutes
Add all ingredients in your Electric Pressure Cooker. Seal the lid and adjust the steam release handle. Cook on High Pressure for 20 minutes. Release the steam naturally, for about 5 minutes.

Flavorful Vegetable Mix

INGREDIENTS for Servings: 2-4

1 small head broccoli, broken into florets	1 cup water
	16 asparagus, trimmed
1 small head cauliflower, broken into florets	5 ounces green beans
	2 carrots, peeled and cut on bias
	Salt to taste

DIRECTIONS and Cooking Time: 15 Minutes
Add water and set trivet on top of water and place steamer basket on top. In an even layer, spread green beans, broccoli, cauliflower, asparagus, and carrots in the steamer basket. Seal the lid and cook on Steam for 3 minutes on High. Release the pressure quickly. Remove basket from the pot and season with salt.

Indian Coconut Kale Curry

INGREDIENTS for Servings: 4

1 can unsweetened coconut cream	¼ cup curry powder
1 package dry onion soup mix	1 large yellow bell pepper, cut into strips
2 cups kale, rinsed and shredded	1 cup cilantro for garnish

DIRECTIONS and Cooking Time: 4 Minutes
Place all ingredients in the Electric Pressure Cooker. Stir the contents and close the lid. Close the lid and press the Manual button. Adjust the cooking time to 4 minutes. Do quick pressure release. Once the lid is open, garnish with cilantro.

Sumac Red Potatoes

INGREDIENTS for Servings: 4

2 tbsp butter	2 tbsp sumac
1 lb red potatoes, cut into wedges	Salt and black pepper to taste

DIRECTIONS and Cooking Time: 25 Minutes
Melt the butter in your Electric Pressure Cooker on Sauté. Mix the potatoes, sumac, and ½ cup of water and seal the lid. Select Manual and cook for 6 minutes on High pressure. Once ready, perform a quick pressure release and unlock the lid. Sprinkle with salt and pepper. Serve immediately.

Indian Dhal With Veggies

INGREDIENTS for Servings: 4

10 oz lentils, soaked overnight	¼ tbsp parsley, chopped
2 tbsp almond butter	½ tbsp chili powder
1 carrot, peeled, chopped	2 tbsp ground cumin
1 potato, peeled, chopped	1 tbsp garam masala
	3 cups vegetable stock
1 bay leaf	Salt to taste

DIRECTIONS and Cooking Time: 35 Minutes
Melt almond butter on Sauté. Add carrots, potatoes, and parsley. Give it a good stir and cook for 10 minutes. Add the remaining ingredients, except for the parsley and press Cancel. If the mixture is very thick, add a bit of water. Seal the lid, select manual and cook on High Pressure for 15 minutes. Once the timer goes off, do a quick release. Serve hot sprinkled with parsley.

Elegant Farro With Greens & Pine Nuts

INGREDIENTS for Servings: 6

6 oz kale, chopped	6 oz spinach, chopped
6 oz collard greens, chopped	1 ½ cups farro
3 oz Swiss chard, chopped	4 tbsp olive oil
	5 cups vegetable broth
3 oz parsley leaves,	1 tbsp salt

chopped 1 medium-sized leek, chopped	½ cup toasted pine nuts

DIRECTIONS and Cooking Time: 15 Minutes
Add farro and vegetable broth to the Electric Pressure Cooker. Season with salt and seal the lid. Cook on Rice mode for 9 minutes on High. Do a quick release and open the lid. Remove farro and wipe the Electric Pressure Cooker clean. Pour two cups of water, insert the steamer basket and place the chopped collard greens on the basket. Seal the lid. Cook on Steam mode for 2 minutes on High. Do a quick release and remove the greens to a large bowl. Toss in the farro, drizzle with olive oil and sprinkle with pine nuts to serve.

Pumpkin Puree
INGREDIENTS for Servings: 4-6

2 lbs small-sized sugar pumpkin, halved and seeds scooped out	1 + ¼ cup water Salt to taste, optional

DIRECTIONS and Cooking Time: 30 Minutes
Prepare the Electric Pressure Cooker by adding 1 cup of water to the pot and placing the steam rack in it. Place the pumpkin halves on the rack. Close and lock the lid. Select MANUAL and cook at HIGH pressure for 14 minutes. When the timer goes off, use a Quick Release. Carefully open the lid. Transfer the pumpkin to a plate and let it cool. Then scoop out the flesh into a bowl. Add ¼ cup of water. Using an immersion blender or food processor, blend until puree. Season with salt and serve.

Buttery Mashed Cauliflower
INGREDIENTS for Servings: 4

2 cups water 1 head cauliflower Celery salt and black pepper to taste	1 tbsp butter ¼ cup heavy cream 1 tbsp fresh parsley, chopped

DIRECTIONS and Cooking Time: 15 Minutes
Into the pot, add water and set trivet on top. Lay cauliflower head onto the trivet. Seal the lid and cook for 8 minutes on High Pressure. Release the pressure quickly. Remove trivet and drain the liquid from the pot. Take back the cauliflower to the pot alongside the pepper, heavy cream, salt and butter. Use an immersion blender to blend until smooth. Top with parsley and serve.

Egg & Ham Traybake
INGREDIENTS for Servings: 4

2 tbsp olive oil 2 shallots, chopped ½ lb ham, chopped	½ cup flour 1 cup feta cheese 1 cup fontina cheese

8 large eggs, beaten 1 cup canned black beans, rinsed	2 tbsp cilantro, chopped ½ cup green onions

DIRECTIONS and Cooking Time: 30 Minutes
Warm the olive oil in your Electric Pressure Cooker on Sauté. Add in shallots and cook for 2-3 minutes. Stir in ham and cook for 3-4 minutes more. In a bowl, whisk eggs with flour and pour over the ham. Top with beans, feta cheese, and fontina cheese. Seal the lid, select Manual, and cook for 15 minutes on High pressure. When over, allow a natural release for 10 minutes and unlock the lid. Scatter with cilantro and green onions. Serve chilled.

Savory Spinach And Leek Relish
INGREDIENTS for Servings: 4

½ lb leeks, chopped 3 cups spinach, chopped 2 ½ cups stock 2 cloves garlic, crushed	½ cup onions, chopped 1 tbsp dry sage 2 tbsp olive oil 1 tbsp nutmeg Salt and black pepper to taste

DIRECTIONS and Cooking Time: 20 Minutes
Heat olive oil and fry leeks for 5 minutes on Sauté. Add in garlic and onions, and cook for 2 minutes. Add the rest of the ingredients and seal the lid. Select Manual and cook for 5 minutes at High. Do a quick release the pressure. Serve.

Spicy Vegetable Salsa
INGREDIENTS for Servings: 4

1 tablespoon olive oil 1 onion, diced 1 cup potatoes, diced ½ cup carrots, diced ½ cup bell pepper, diced 1 cup vegetable broth ½ teaspoon ground cumin	2 cans diced tomatoes ½ teaspoon kosher salt ¼ teaspoon chili powder 1 cup salsa 2 cups shredded cheese ½ cup milk

DIRECTIONS and Cooking Time: 12 Minutes
Add the oil and onion into the Electric Pressure Cooker and "Sauté" for 3 minutes. Stir in all the vegetables and 'sauté' for another 5 minutes. Add the remaining ingredients, except the salsa, to the pot and secure the lid. Select 'manual' setting and cook at high pressure for 4 minutes. After the beep, 'Quick release' the steam and remove the lid. Stir in the salsa and serve hot.

Parsnips & Cauliflower Mash
INGREDIENTS for Servings: 2

½ lb parsnips, peeled and cubed ¼ head cauliflower, cut into florets 1 garlic cloves Salt and pepper to taste	½ cup water 2 tbsp sour cream 2 tbsp grated Parmesan cheese ½ tbsp butter ½ tbsp minced chives

DIRECTIONS and Cooking Time: 15 Minutes
In the pot, mix parsnips, garlic, water, salt, cauliflower, and pepper. Seal the lid and cook on High Pressure for 4 minutes. Release the pressure quickly. Drain parsnips and cauliflower and return to pot. Add Parmesan, butter, and sour cream. Use a potato masher to mash until desired consistency is attained. Into the mashed parsnip, add a half of the chives; place to a serving plate and garnish with remaining chives.

Feta & Nut Green Beans
INGREDIENTS for Servings: 2

Juice from ½ lemon 1 cup water ½ cup green beans, trimmed ⅓ cup chopped toasted pine nuts	⅓ cup feta cheese, crumbled 2 tbsp olive oil Salt and black pepper to taste

DIRECTIONS and Cooking Time: 15 Minutes
Add water and set the rack over the water and the steamer basket on the rack. Loosely heap green beans into the steamer basket. Seal lid and cook on High Pressure for 5 minutes. Release pressure quickly. Drop green beans into a salad bowl. Top with the olive oil, feta cheese, pepper, and pine nuts.

Meat Lover's Omelet
INGREDIENTS for Servings: 6

10 beaten eggs 3 sausage links, sliced 1 onion, diced 1 tsp garlic powder Salt and black pepper to taste	3 bacon slices, cooked ½ cup smoked sliced ham ½ cup shredded cheddar cheese

DIRECTIONS and Cooking Time: 25 Minutes
Beat eggs in a bowl. Stir in sausages, onion, salt, garlic powder, and pepper. Pour in a greased baking pan and cover with aluminum foil. Pour 1 cup of water in your Electric Pressure Cooker and fit in a trivet. Place the pan on top of the trivet. Seal the lid, select Manual, and cook for 15 minutes on High pressure. Once done, allow a natural release for 10 minutes and unlock the lid. Remove the foil and scatter with cooked bacon, smoked ham, and cheddar cheese. Broil for 4-6 minutes until the cheese is melt. Serve hot!

Beets And Cheese
INGREDIENTS for Servings: 4-6

6 medium beets, trimmed Salt and ground black pepper to taste	1 cup water ¼ cup cheese (by choice), crumbled

DIRECTIONS and Cooking Time: 30 Minutes
Pour the water into the Electric Pressure Cooker and insert a steamer basket. Place the beets in the basket. Close and lock the lid. Select MANUAL and cook at HIGH pressure for 20 minutes. Once cooking is complete, let the pressure Release Naturally for 10 minutes. Release any remaining steam manually. Uncover the pot. Transfer the beets to a bowl and let them cool. Season with salt and pepper and add the blue cheese. Serve.

Indian Lentils Dhal
INGREDIENTS for Servings: 2-4

10 oz lentils, soaked overnight 2 tbsp almond butter 1 carrot, peeled, chopped 1 potato, peeled, chopped 1 bay leaf	¼ tbsp parsley, chopped ½ tbsp chili powder 2 tbsp ground cumin 1 tbsp garam masala 3 cups vegetable stock Salt to taste

DIRECTIONS and Cooking Time: 35 Minutes
Melt almond butter on Sauté. Add carrots, potatoes, and parsley. Give it a good stir and cook for 10 minutes. Press Cancel and add the remaining ingredients. Cook on High Pressure for 15 minutes. Do a quick release and serve hot.

Cauliflower Salad With Mozzarella Cheese
INGREDIENTS for Servings: 3

1 pound cauliflower florets 2 bell peppers, thinly sliced 1 red onion, thinly sliced 1/2 cup fresh flat-leaf parsley, coarsely chopped 1/4 cup green olives, pitted and coarsely chopped	1/4 cup extra-virgin olive oil 2 tablespoons fresh lime juice 1 teaspoon hot mustard Sea salt and ground black pepper, to taste 4 ounces mozzarella cheese, crumbled

DIRECTIONS and Cooking Time: 10 Minutes
Add 1 cup of water and steamer basket to the inner pot. Place the cauliflower in the steamer basket. Secure the lid. Choose the "Steam" mode and cook for 2 minutes at High pressure. Once cooking is complete,

use a quick pressure release; carefully remove the lid. Toss the cooked cauliflower with peppers, onion, parsley, and olives. In a small bowl, prepare the salad dressing by mixing the olive oil, lime juice, mustard, salt, and black pepper. Dress your salad and serve garnished with the crumbled mozzarella cheese. Bon appétit!

Mom's Carrots With Walnuts & Berries

INGREDIENTS for Servings: 4

2 lb carrots, cut into rounds	¼ cup dried cranberries
½ cup walnuts, chopped	Salt and black pepper to taste
1 tbsp butter	1 tbsp vinegar

DIRECTIONS and Cooking Time: 15 Minutes
Select Sauté and melt the butter. Add in carrots and cook for 5 minutes until tender. Add cranberries, 1 cup of water, and salt. Seal the lid, press Manual, and cook for 3 minutes at High. When done, do a quick pressure release. Pour in the vinegar, and black pepper, and give it a good stir. Scatter the walnuts over and serve.

Poblano Pepper & Sweet Corn Side Dish

INGREDIENTS for Servings: 6

1 tbsp vegetable oil	¾ cup sliced red onions
½ cup heavy whipping cream	4 poblano peppers, sliced
1 tsp cumin, ground	6 tbsp sour cream
Salt and black pepper to taste	2 tbsp lemon juice
½ cup frozen corn	

DIRECTIONS and Cooking Time: 23 Minutes
Heat oil on Sauté. Add the peppers, skin side facing down, and onions. Cook for 8 minutes. In a mixing bowl, add heavy cream, sour cream, and lemon juice. Mix well. Stir in the peppers, add in the corn and ¼ cup of water. Cook for 5 minutes. Season with salt and pepper, and sprinkle with ground cumin to serve.

Broccoli Leeks Green Soup

INGREDIENTS for Servings: 2-4

2 tbsp olive oil	1 cup green beans
1 head broccoli, cut into florets	2 cups vegetable broth
4 celery stalks, chopped thinly	3 whole black peppercorns
1 leek, chopped thinly	Salt to taste
1 zucchini, chopped	Water to cover
	2 cups chopped kale

DIRECTIONS and Cooking Time: 30 Minutes
Add broccoli, leek, beans, salt, peppercorns, zucchini, and celery. Mix in vegetable broth, oil, and water. Seal the lid and cook on High Pressure for 4 minutes. Release pressure naturally for 5 minutes, then release the remaining pressure quickly. Stir in kale; set on Sauté, and cook until tender.

Asparagus And Mushrooms

INGREDIENTS for Servings: 4

1 lb. asparagus spears, trimmed	Salt and pepper, to taste
2 garlic cloves, minced	½ cup fresh mushrooms
¼ cup water	1 tbsp. coconut oil

DIRECTIONS and Cooking Time: 5 Minutes
Press the Sauté button on the Electric Pressure Cooker and heat the oil. Add the garlic and sauté for 2 or 3 minutes until fragrant. Add the asparagus spears and mushrooms. Add salt and pepper and add the water. Lock the lid. Set the Electric Pressure Cooker to Manual mode, then set the timer for 5 minutes at High Pressure. Once cooking is complete, do a quick pressure release. Carefully open the lid. Serve warm.

Quick Indian Creamy Eggplant

INGREDIENTS for Servings: 6

4 cups eggplants, chopped	1 onion, thinly sliced
¼ tsp turmeric, ground	¼ tsp cayenne pepper
¼ tsp garam masala	¼ cup heavy cream
1 tomato, chopped	¼ tsp goda masala
½ tsp peanut oil	Salt and black pepper to taste

DIRECTIONS and Cooking Time: 30 Minutes
Grease a baking dish with peanut oil. Add tomato and onion, then place the eggplants on top of them. Sprinkle with turmeric, black pepper, salt, goda masala, garam masala, and cayenne; do not stir. Top with heavy cream. Pour 1 cup of water in the IP and insert a trivet. Put the dish on the trivet. Seal the lid, press Manual, and cook at High for 10 minutes. Do a quick pressure release and serve.

Steamed Artichokes & Green Beans With Mayo Dip

INGREDIENTS for Servings: 4

4 artichokes, trimmed	1 tbsp lemon juice
½ pound green beans, trimmed	½ cup mayonnaise
1 lemon, halved	1 cup water
1 tbsp lemon zest	Salt to taste
3 cloves garlic, crushed	1 handful of parsley, chopped

DIRECTIONS and Cooking Time: 20 Minutes

Rub the artichokes and green beans with lemon. Add water into the pot. Set steamer rack over water and set steamer basket on top. Place artichokes and green beans into the basket and sprinkle with salt. Seal lid and cook on high Pressure for 10 minutes. Release the pressure quickly. In a mixing bowl, combine mayonnaise, garlic, lemon juice, and lemon zest. Season to taste with salt. Serve with warm steamed artichokes and green beans sprinkled with parsley.

Creamy Spinach Tagliatelle With Mushrooms

INGREDIENTS for Servings: 4

8 oz spinach tagliatelle	¼ cup grated Parmesan cheese
6 oz frozen mixed mushrooms	2 garlic cloves, crushed
3 tbsp butter, unsalted	¼ cup heavy cream
¼ cup feta cheese	1 tbsp Italian seasoning mix

DIRECTIONS and Cooking Time: 25 Minutes
Melt butter on Sauté, and stir-fry the garlic for a minute. Stir in feta, Italian seasoning, and mushrooms. Add tagliatelle, 2 cups of water, and heavy cream. Cook on High Pressure for 4 minutes. Quick release the pressure and top with parmesan.

Easy Homemade Pizza

INGREDIENTS for Servings: 2-4

1 pizza crust	½ cup grated gouda cheese
½ cup tomato paste	2 tbsp extra virgin olive oil
¼ cup water	
1 tsp sugar	12 olives
1 tsp dried oregano	1 cup arugula for serving
4 oz button mushrooms, chopped	

DIRECTIONS and Cooking Time: 20 Minutes
Grease the bottom of a baking dish with one tablespoon of olive oil. Line some parchment paper. Flour the working surface and roll out the pizza dough to the approximate size of your Electric Pressure Cooker. gently fit the dough in the previously prepared baking dish. In a bowl, combine tomato paste, water, sugar, and dry oregano. Spread the mixture over dough, make a layer with button mushrooms and grated gouda. Add a trivet inside the pot and pour in 1 cup of water. Seal the lid, and cook for 15 minutes on High Pressure. Do a quick release. Remove the pizza from your pot using a parchment paper. Sprinkle with the remaining olive oil and top with olives and arugula. Cut and serve.

Creamy Artichoke, Garlic, And Zucchini

INGREDIENTS for Servings: 12

2 tablespoons coconut oil	2 medium zucchinis, sliced
1 bulb garlic, minced	½ cup whipping cream
1 large artichoke hearts, cleaned and sliced	½ cup vegetable broth
	Salt and pepper

DIRECTIONS and Cooking Time: 10 Minutes
Press the Sauté button and heat the oil Sauté the garlic until fragrant. Add the rest of the ingredients. Stir the contents and close the lid. Close the lid and press the Manual button. Adjust the cooking time to 10 minutes. Do quick pressure release.

Steamed Artichokes With Mayo Dip

INGREDIENTS for Servings: 3

1 cup water	1/2 cup mayonnaise
1 bay leaf	1 teaspoon garlic, pressed
1 lemon wedge	
3 medium artichokes, trimmed	2 tablespoons fresh parsley, minced
Sea salt, to taste	

DIRECTIONS and Cooking Time: 20 Minutes
Place water and bay leaf in the inner pot. Rub the lemon wedge all over the outside of the prepared artichokes. Season them with salt. Place the artichokes in the steamer basket; lower the steamer basket into the inner pot. Secure the lid. Choose the "Manual" mode and cook for 11 minutes at High pressure. Once cooking is complete, use a quick pressure release; carefully remove the lid. Meanwhile, mix the mayonnaise with the garlic and parsley. Serve the artichokes with the mayo dip on the side. Bon appétit!

Lime & Ginger Eggplants

INGREDIENTS for Servings: 2

2 eggplants, chopped	1 tsp paprika
2 tsp minced ginger	1 tsp cumin
1 onion, chopped	1 tsp cilantro
½ lime, zested and juiced	1 tsp turmeric
	Salt and black pepper to taste
1 tbsp tomato paste	
2 tbsp olive oil	¾ cup vegetable broth

DIRECTIONS and Cooking Time: 25 Minutes
Heat oil on Sauté and cook onion, ginger, and eggplants for 5 minutes. Add in remaining ingredients. Seal the lid, press Manual, and cook for 10 minutes at High. After cooking, do a quick pressure release.

Palak Paneer

INGREDIENTS for Servings: 6

1 ½ cups paneer cubes	1 yellow onion, chopped
½ cup whipping cream	½ jalapeño pepper, chopped
Salt and black pepper to taste	1 tbsp fresh ginger, chopped
1 tsp ground turmeric	5 cloves garlic, chopped
2 tsp garam masala	2 tsp olive oil
½ tsp cayenne pepper	
2 tsp ground cumin	
2 tomatoes, chopped	
1 lb spinach, chopped	

DIRECTIONS and Cooking Time: 23 Minutes
Place your IP on Sauté and heat the oil. Add in jalapeño, garlic, and ginger and sauté for 3 minutes. Add in the remaining ingredients, except for whipping cream. Pour 1 cup of water, seal the lid, press Manual, and cook at High for 10 minutes. When ready, do a quick release and allow to cool down a bit. Puree the mixture using an immersion blender. Gently stir in the paneer. Serve warm, topped with a dollop of whipping cream.

Tomato & Apple Cider Infused Ratatouille

INGREDIENTS for Servings: 4

1 eggplant, sliced	1 zucchini, sliced
1 cup tomatoes, crushed	1 purple onion, chopped
3 Roma tomatoes, sliced	¼ tsp chili powder
¼ tsp apple cider vinegar	Salt and black pepper to taste
1 tbsp olive oil	1 tsp garlic, minced

DIRECTIONS and Cooking Time: 45 Minutes
Put a trivet in the IP and pour in 1 cup of water. Place a baking dish over the trivet. Add a layer of crushed tomatoes at the bottom of the dish. Add the eggplant, garlic, salt, pepper, chili powder, onion, zucchini, olive oil, apple cider vinegar, roma tomatoes. Top with a layer of the remaining crushed tomatoes. Seal the lid and press Manual. Cook at High for 20 minutes. After cooking, do a natural pressure release for 10 minutes.

Power Green Minestrone Stew With Lemon

INGREDIENTS for Servings: 4

1 head cauliflower, in florets	1 tsp olive oil
2 green bell peppers, sliced	4 cups vegetable broth
2 celery stalks, chopped	1 bunch kale, chopped
1 tsp garlic, minced	2 tsp fresh lemon juice
4 spring onions, chopped	Salt and black pepper to taste
	Grated Grana Padano

DIRECTIONS and Cooking Time: 35 Minutes
Heat the oil on Sauté. Cook the spring onions and garlic until tender, for about 2 minutes. Add the remaining ingredients, except for the kale and Grana Padano cheese. Seal the lid, press Manual and cook for 10 minutes at High. Once the cooking is over, do a quick release. Add in the kale. Place the lid and cook for 12-15 minutes until tender on Sauté, stirring occasionally. Divide between 4 bowls and serve sprinkled with Grana Padano cheese.

Easy Vegan Pizza

INGREDIENTS for Servings: 2

1½ cups water	½ cup vegan cheese, shredded
1 pizza crust, store-bought	1 tsp oregano, chopped
¼ cup vegan Alfred sauce	

DIRECTIONS and Cooking Time: 20 Minutes
Prepare the Electric Pressure Cooker by adding the water to the pot and placing the steam rack in it. Line a baking dish that can fit into the pot with parchment paper. Place the pizza crust inside the baking dish and spread the Alfredo sauce over. Sprinkle the cheese over the crust and top with oregano. Put the baking dish on the rack. Secure the lid. Select MANUAL and cook at HIGH pressure for 5 minutes. When the timer beeps, use a Quick Release. Carefully unlock the lid. Serve.

Vegetarian Chipotle Stew

INGREDIENTS for Servings: 2

½ cup canned diced tomatoes	½ tbsp chili powder
⅓ cup cashews, chopped	1 tsp salt
¼ cup onion, chopped	3 cups water
¼ cup red lentils	½ cup carrots, chopped
¼ cup red quinoa	¼ cup canned black beans, rinsed and drained
1 chipotle pepper, chopped	2 tbsp fresh parsley, chopped
1 garlic clove, minced	

DIRECTIONS and Cooking Time: 45 Minutes
In the pot, mix tomatoes, onion, chipotle pepper, chili powder, lentils, walnuts, carrots, quinoa, garlic, and salt. Stir in more water. Seal the lid, Press Soup/Stew and cook for 30 minutes on High Pressure. Release the pressure quickly. Into the chili, add black beans; simmer on Sauté until heated through. Add ¼ cup to 1 cup water if you want a thinner consistency. Top with a garnish of parsley.

Arabic-style Cauliflower Salad

INGREDIENTS for Servings: 3

2 cups cauliflower rice	½ cup parsley
4 tbsp sesame oil	1 tsp nutmeg
½ cup spring onions, chopped	½ cup mint
	1 tsp garlic, minced
½ cucumber, diced	1 cup tomato puree
3 tbsp lime juice	Salt and black pepper to taste

DIRECTIONS and Cooking Time: 10 Minutes
Heat a tablespoon of sesame oil in the pressure cooker on Sauté. Add garlic and cook for a minute. Add tomato puree and cauli rice, and sauté them for 2-3 minutes. Transfer to a bowl. Add the remaining ingredients to the bowl and give the mixture a good stir to combine well. Divide among 3 Servings bowls.

Delicious Mushroom Goulash

INGREDIENTS for Servings: 4

6 oz portobello mushrooms, sliced	2 potatoes, chopped
1 cup green peas	1 tbsp apple cider vinegar
1 cup pearl onions, minced	1 tbsp rosemary
2 carrots, chopped	Salt and black pepper to taste
½ cup celery stalks, chopped	2 tbsp butter
2 garlic cloves, crushed	4 cups vegetable stock

DIRECTIONS and Cooking Time: 45 Minutes
Melt butter on Sauté and stir-fry onions, carrots, celery stalks, and garlic, for 2-3 minutes. Season with salt, pepper, and rosemary. Add the remaining ingredients and seal the lid. Cook on High Pressure for 30 minutes. When ready, release the pressure naturally, for about 5 minutes.

Lentil & Carrot Chili

INGREDIENTS for Servings: 2-4

1 tbsp olive oil	1 onion, chopped
1 onion, chopped	4 carrots, halved lengthwise
1 cup celery, chopped	
2 garlic cloves, chopped	1 tbsp harissa, or more to taste
3 cups vegetable stock	½ tsp sea salt
1½ cups dried lentils, rinsed	A handful of fresh parsley, chopped

DIRECTIONS and Cooking Time: 30 Minutes
Warm olive oil on Sauté. Add in onion, garlic, and celery, and Sauté for 5 minutes until onion is soft. Mix in lentils, carrots, and vegetable stock. Seal the lid and cook on High Pressure for 10 minutes. Release the pressure quickly. Mix lentils with salt and harissa and serve topped with parsley.

Electric Pressure Cooker Cauliflower Curry

INGREDIENTS for Servings: 4

2 cups cauliflower florets	1 can full-fat coconut milk
2 tablespoon garam masala	Salt and pepper to taste
2 cups water	

DIRECTIONS and Cooking Time: 4 Minutes
Place all ingredients in the Electric Pressure Cooker. Stir the contents and close the lid. Close the lid and press the Manual button. Adjust the cooking time to 4 minutes. Do quick pressure release.

Carrot Vegan Gazpacho

INGREDIENTS for Servings: 2-4

1 pound trimmed carrots	2 tbsp lemon juice
A pinch of salt	1 red onion, chopped
1 pound tomatoes, chopped	2 cloves garlic
	2 tbsp white wine vinegar
1 cucumber, peeled and chopped	Salt and ground black pepper to taste
¼ cup olive oil	

DIRECTIONS and Cooking Time: 2 Hours 30 Minutes
Add carrots, salt and enough water. Seal the lid and cook for 20 minutes on High Pressure. Do a quick release. Set the beets to a bowl and place in the refrigerator to cool. In a blender, add carrots, cucumber, red onion, pepper, garlic, oil, tomatoes, lemon juice, vinegar, and salt. Blend until very smooth. Place gazpacho to a serving bowl, chill while covered for 2 hours.

Electric Pressure Cooker Steamed Artichoke

INGREDIENTS for Servings: 8

2 cups water	1 tablespoon peppercorns
2 lemons, one sliced and one juiced	3 cloves of garlic, minced
6 artichokes, cleaned and trimmed	2 cups olive oil

DIRECTIONS and Cooking Time: 5 Minutes
Pour the water and juice from one lemon in the pressure cooker. Place the artichokes, peppercorns, garlic and olive oil in the pressure cooker Close the lid and press the Manual button.4. Adjust the cooking time to 5 minutes. Do quick pressure release.

English Vegetable Potage

INGREDIENTS for Servings: 4

1 lb potatoes, peeled, cut into bite-sized pieces	A handful of fresh celery leaves
2 carrots, peeled, chopped	2 tbsp butter, unsalted
3 celery stalks, chopped	3 tbsp olive oil
2 onions, peeled, chopped	2 cups vegetable broth
1 zucchini, chopped into ½-inch thick slices	1 tbsp paprika
	Salt and black pepper to taste
	2 bay leaves

DIRECTIONS and Cooking Time: 50 Minutes
Warm olive oil on Sauté and stir-fry the onions for 3-4 minutes, until translucent. Add carrots, celery, zucchini, and ¼ cup of broth. Continue to cook for 10 more minutes, stirring constantly. Stir in potatoes, paprika, salt, pepper, bay leaves, remaining broth, and celery leaves. Seal the lid and cook on Meat/Stew mode for 30 minutes on High. Do a quick release and stir in butter.

Veggie Flax Patties

INGREDIENTS for Servings: 4

2 tbsp canola oil	Salt and black pepper to taste
1 bag frozen mixed veggies	1 tbsp cumin
1 cup cauliflower florets	1 cup flax meal

DIRECTIONS and Cooking Time: 30 Minutes
Pour 1 cup of water in your IP. Combine mixed veggies and cauliflower florets in a steamer basket and then lower the basket inside the pot. Seal the lid, select Manual and cook for 5 minutes at High. After the timer goes off, do a quick pressure release. Transfer the veggies to a bowl and discard the water. Mash the veggies with a potato masher, add cumin and allow them to cool for 10 minutes. When safe to handle, stir in the flax meal and shape the mixture into 4 equal patties. Wipe the pot clean and add canola oil. Set to Sauté. Add veggie burgers, and cook for 6 minutes, flipping once halfway through cooking. Serve.

Steamed Artichoke With Garlic Mayo Sauce

INGREDIENTS for Servings: 2-4

2 large artichokes	½ cup mayonnaise
2 cups water	Salt and black pepper to taste
2 garlic cloves, smashed	Juice of 1 lime

DIRECTIONS and Cooking Time: 20 Minutes
Using a serrated knife, trim about 1 inch from the artichokes' top. Into the pot, add water and set trivet over. Lay the artichokes on the trivet. Seal lid and cook for 14 minutes on High Pressure. Release the pressure quickly. Mix the mayonnaise with garlic and lime juice. Season with salt and pepper. Serve artichokes in a platter with garlic mayo on the side.

Steamed Vegetables Side Dish

INGREDIENTS for Servings: 6

2 bell peppers, sliced	1 teaspoon Italian seasoning
2 large zucchinis, sliced	2 tablespoon olive oil
½ cup peeled garlic cloves	¼ cup parmesan cheese, grated
Salt and pepper to taste	

DIRECTIONS and Cooking Time: 10 Minutes
Place a trivet or steamer in the Electric Pressure Cooker and pour a cup of water. In a baking dish that will fit inside the Electric Pressure Cooker, mix the pepper, zucchini, and garlic. Season with salt, pepper, and Italian seasoning. Pour in olive oil and toss to combine. Add the parmesan cheese on top. Place on top of the steamer basket. Close the lid and press the Steam button. Adjust the cooking time to 10 minutes. Do quick pressure release.

Carrot & Chickpea Boil With Cherry Tomatoes

INGREDIENTS for Servings: 4

1 cup chickpeas, cooked	2 carrots, chopped
1 onion, peeled, chopped	2 garlic cloves, crushed
A handful of string beans, trimmed	4 cherry tomatoes
1 apple, chopped into 1-inch cubes	A handful of fresh mint
½ cup raisins	1 tbsp grated ginger
½ tbsp button mushrooms, chopped	½ cup freshly squeezed orange juice
	½ tbsp salt

DIRECTIONS and Cooking Time: 20 Minutes
Place all ingredients in the Electric Pressure Cooker. Pour enough water to cover. Cook on High Pressure for 8 minutes. Do a natural release, for 10 minutes.

Sage Cauliflower Mash

INGREDIENTS for Servings: 2-4

2 cups water	1 tbsp fresh sage, chopped
1 head cauliflower	½ tsp ground black pepper
1 tbsp butter	
¼ tsp celery salt	
¼ cup heavy cream	

DIRECTIONS and Cooking Time: 15 Minutes
Into the pot, add water and set trivet on top. Lay cauliflower head onto the trivet. Seal the lid and cook for 8 minutes on High Pressure. Release the pressure quickly. Remove trivet and Drain the liquid from the pot. Take back the cauliflower to the pot alongside the pepper, heavy cream, salt and butter. Use an immersion blender to blend until smooth. Top with sage and serve.

Parmesan Lentil Spread

INGREDIENTS for Servings: 2

1 cup lentils, cooked	1 tbsp tomato paste
⅓ cup sweet corn	Salt to taste
1 tomato, diced	¼ tsp red pepper flakes
¼ tsp dried oregano, ground	1 tbsp olive oil
½ tbsp Parmesan cheese	⅓ cup water
	2 tbsp red wine

DIRECTIONS and Cooking Time: 15 Minutes
Heat oil on Sauté and add tomatoes, tomato paste, and half of the water. Sprinkle with salt and oregano and stir-fry for 5 minutes. Press Cancel and add lentils, sweet corn, and wine. Pour in the remaining water and seal the lid. Cook on High Pressure for 2 minutes. Do a quick release. Set aside to cool completely and refrigerate for 30 minutes. Sprinkle with Parmesan Cheese before serving.

Parmesan & Veggie Mash

INGREDIENTS for Servings: 2

1 pound yukon gold potato, chopped	2 tbsp butter, melted
½ cup cauliflower, broken into florets	2 tbsp milk
	Salt to taste
⅓ carrot, chopped	1 garlic clove, minced
⅓ cup Parmesan cheese, shredded	Fresh parsley for garnish

DIRECTIONS and Cooking Time: 15 Minutes
Into the pot, add veggies, salt and cover with enough water. Seal the lid and cook on High Pressure for 10 minutes. Release the pressure quickly. Drain the vegetables and mash them with a potato masher. Add garlic, butter and milk, and Whisk until everything is well incorporated. Serve topped with Parmesan cheese and chopped parsley.

Potato Spinach Corn Mix

INGREDIENTS for Servings: 6

1 tablespoon olive oil	1 cup vegetable stock
3 scallions, chopped	2 tablespoons light soy sauce
½ cup onion, chopped	
2 large white potatoes, peeled and diced1 tablespoon ginger, grated	2 large cloves of garlic, diced
	⅓ teaspoon white pepper1 teaspoon salt
3 cups frozen corn kernels	3-4 handfuls of baby spinach leaves
1 tablespoon fish sauce	Juice of ½ lemon

DIRECTIONS and Cooking Time: 10 Minutes
Put the oil, ginger, garlic and onions in the Electric Pressure Cooker and 'sauté' for 5 minutes. Add all the remaining ingredients except the spinach leaves and lime juice Secure the lid and cook on the 'manual' setting for 5 minutes at high pressure. After the beep, 'Quick release' the steam and remove the lid.5. Add the spinach and cook for 3 minutes on 'sauté' Drizzle the lime juice over the dish and serve hot.

Electric Pressure Cooker Basic Steamed Vegetables

INGREDIENTS for Servings: 4

2 bell peppers, cut into large slices	1 tablespoon Italian herb mix
3 small zucchinis, cut into thick slices	2 tablespoon olive oil
½ cup peeled garlic, minced	

DIRECTIONS and Cooking Time: 7 Minutes
Place all ingredients in a mixing bowl. Season with salt if desired and toss to coat everything. Place a trivet in the Electric Pressure Cooker and pour 1 cup of water. Place the vegetables on the steamer. Close the lid and press the Steam button. Adjust the cooking time to 7 minutes. Do quick pressure release.

Cabbage With Carrot

INGREDIENTS for Servings: 2-4

2 tbsp coconut oil	1 head cabbage, shredded
2 small onions, sliced	2 carrots, sliced
2 cloves garlic, chopped	1 cup water
Salt to taste	2 tbsp fresh lemon juice
1 tbsp curry powder	
1 jalapeño pepper, deseeded and chopped	½ cup desiccated unsweetened coconut

DIRECTIONS and Cooking Time: 35 Minutes
Select the SAUTÉ setting on the Electric Pressure Cooker and heat the oil. Add the onion and sauté for about 4 minutes, until softened. Add the garlic, salt, curry powder, and jalapeño pepper, stir and sauté for 1 minute more. Add the cabbage, carrots, water, lemon juice, and coconut. Press the CANCEL key to stop the SAUTÉ function. Close and lock the lid. Select MANUAL and cook at HIGH pressure for 5 minutes. Once cooking is complete, use a Natural Release for 10 minutes, then release any remaining

pressure manually. Open the lid. Taste for seasoning and add more salt if needed. Serve.

Pure Basmati Rice Meal

INGREDIENTS for Servings: 4

1 cup chopped cauliflower	1 small onion, sliced
¼ cup chopped green onions	1 cup basmati rice
	1 tsp. olive oil

DIRECTIONS and Cooking Time: 10 Minutes
Purée the cauliflower until smooth in a blender and set aside. Press the Sauté bottom on the Electric Pressure Cooker. Grease the pot with olive oil. Add the onions and sauté for 3 minutes until translucent and softened. Add the cauliflower purée, rice and green onions. Lock the lid. Set the Electric Pressure Cooker to Manual mode, then set the timer for 4 minutes at Low Pressure. Once cooking is complete, do a natural pressure release. Carefully open the lid. Transfer the cooked recipe on serving plates. Serve warm.

Cauliflower & Potato Curry With Cilantro

INGREDIENTS for Servings: 4

1 tbsp vegetable oil	1 onion, minced
1 head cauliflower, cored and cut into florets	1 jalapeño pepper, deseeded and minced
1 potato, peeled and diced	1 tbsp curry paste
1 tbsp ghee	1 tbsp ground turmeric
2 tbsp cumin seeds	½ tsp chili pepper
4 garlic cloves, minced	1 cup water
1 tomato, cored and chopped	Salt and black pepper to taste
	A handful of cilantro leaves, chopped

DIRECTIONS and Cooking Time: 40 Minutes
Warm oil on Sauté mode. Add in potato and cauliflower and cook for 8 to 10 minutes until lightly browned; season with salt. Set the vegetables to a bowl. Add ghee to the pot. Mix in cumin seeds and cook for 10 seconds until they start to pop; add onion and cook for 3 minutes until softened. Mix in garlic; cook for 30 seconds. Add in tomato, curry paste, chili pepper, jalapeño pepper, and turmeric; cook for 4 to 6 minutes. Return potato and cauliflower to the pot. Stir in water. Seal the lid and cook on High Pressure for 4 minutes. Quick release the pressure. Top with cilantro.

Mirin Tofu Bowl

INGREDIENTS for Servings: 6

20 oz smoked tofu, sliced	3 cups cooked brown rice
2 ½ tbsp oyster sauce	1 tsp rosemary
2 tbsp mirin wine	2 tbsp fresh chives, chopped
3 garlic cloves, minced	Salt and black pepper to taste
2 tsp olive oil	1-inch piece of fresh ginger, grated
2 cups vegetable broth	
1 onion, chopped	

DIRECTIONS and Cooking Time: 10 Minutes
Heat oil on Sauté and stir-fry tofu cubes until lightly browned. In a blender, add in the remaining ingredients, except for the rice. Blend until you obtain a smooth paste. Transfer the mixture to the pressure cooker. Select Manual and cook for 2 minutes at High. Do a quick pressure release. Serve on top of cooked rice.

Steamed Paprika Broccoli

INGREDIENTS for Servings: 2

¼ tsp. ground black pepper	1 head broccoli, cut into florets
1 tbsp. freshly squeezed lemon juice	1 tbsp. paprika
¼ tsp. salt	1 cup water

DIRECTIONS and Cooking Time: 6 Minutes
Place a trivet or the steamer rack in the Electric Pressure Cooker and pour in the water. Place the broccoli florets on the trivet and sprinkle salt, pepper, paprika, and lemon juice. Lock the lid. Set the Electric Pressure Cooker to Steam mode, then set the timer for 6 minutes at High Pressure. Once cooking is complete, do a quick pressure release. Carefully open the lid. Serve immediately.

Celery & Red Bean Stew

INGREDIENTS for Servings: 4

6 oz red beans, cooked	1 bay leaf
2 carrots, chopped	2 cups vegetable broth
2 celery stalks, cut into pieces	3 tbsp olive oil
1 onion, peeled, chopped	1 tbsp salt
	A handful of fresh parsley
2 tbsp tomato paste	1 tbsp of flour

DIRECTIONS and Cooking Time: 30 Minutes
Warm olive oil on Sauté and stir-fry the onion, for 3 minutes, until soft. Add celery and carrots. Cook for 5 more minutes, adding 1 tbsp of broth at the time. Add red beans, bay leaf, salt, parsley, and tomato paste. Stir in 1 tbsp of flour and pour in the remaining broth. Seal the lid and cook on High pressure for 5 minutes on. Do a natural release, for about 10 minutes. Sprinkle with some fresh parsley and serve warm.

Spinach & Mushroom Tagliatelle

INGREDIENTS for Servings: 2-4

1 lb spinach tagliatelle	¼ cup grated Parmesan cheese
6 oz frozen mixed mushrooms	2 garlic cloves, crushed
3 tbsp butter, unsalted	¼ cup heavy cream
¼ cup feta cheese	1 tbsp Italian seasoning mix

DIRECTIONS and Cooking Time: 25 Minutes
Melt butter on Sauté, and stir-fry the garlic for a minute. Stir in feta, and mushrooms. Add tagliatelle and 2 cups of water. Cook on High Pressure for 4 minutes. Quick release the pressure and top with parmesan.

Broccoli, Cauliflower & Zucchini Cakes

INGREDIENTS for Servings: 4

1 zucchini, peeled and grated	1 cup veggie broth
3 cups cauliflower florets	½ onion, diced
	½ tsp turmeric powder
1 carrot, grated	2 tbsp olive oil
2 cups broccoli florets	1 tbsp sage
	Salt and black pepper to taste

DIRECTIONS and Cooking Time: 30 Minutes
Heat 1 tbsp olive oil on Sauté and cook onion for 3 minutes. Add carrot and cook for 1 more minute. Pour in broth. Stir in the remaining vegetables, seal the lid, and cook for 5 minutes at High. Do a quick pressure release. Mash veggies with a potato masher and stir in the seasonings. Let cool for a few minutes and make burger patties out of the mixture. On Sauté, heat remaining oil. Cook patties for 4 minutes in total.

Puréed Chili Carrots

INGREDIENTS for Servings: 4

1½ cups water	1½ lbs. carrots, chopped
1 tbsp. maple syrup	
1 tbsp. coconut oil	1 tsp. chili powder

DIRECTIONS and Cooking Time: 5 Minutes
Pour the water into the Electric Pressure Cooker. Place the chopped carrots inside the steamer basket. Arrange the basket in the Electric Pressure Cooker. Lock the lid. Set the Electric Pressure Cooker to Manual mode, then set the timer for 4 minutes on High Pressure. Once cooking is complete, do a quick pressure release. Carefully open the lid. Transfer the carrots along with the remaining ingredients to a food processor. Process until puréed and smooth. Serve immediately!

Vegetable Medley With Brazil Nuts

INGREDIENTS for Servings: 4

¾ cup Brazil nuts, chopped	¾ cup Italian seasoning
½ cup basil, chopped	1/3 cup nutritional yeast
2 garlic cloves, minced	
½ cup olive oil	1 lb grape tomatoes, diced
1 cup vegetable broth	
3 zucchinis, chopped	Salt and black pepper to taste
½ tsp red pepper flakes	3 cups cremini mushrooms, sliced

DIRECTIONS and Cooking Time: 16 Minutes
Heat the olive oil on Sauté and cook zucchini, mushrooms, and garlic for 5 minutes. Add the remaining ingredients, except for the nuts and basil, and stir to combine. Seal the lid, press Manual, and cook for 6 minutes at High. After cooking, do a quick pressure release. Serve hot, sprinkled with basil and topped with nuts.

Sweet Potato Medallions With Garlic & Rosemary

INGREDIENTS for Servings: 4

1 cup water	4 sweet potatoes
1 tbsp fresh rosemary	2 tbsp butter
1 tbsp garlic powder	Salt to taste

DIRECTIONS and Cooking Time: 25 Minutes
Add water and place steamer rack over the water. Use a fork to prick sweet potatoes all over and set onto steamer rack. Seal the lid and cook on High Pressure for 12 minutes. Release the pressure quickly. Transfer sweet potatoes to a cutting board and slice into ½-inch medallions and ensure they are peeled. Melt butter in the on Sauté mode. Add in the medallions and cook each side for 2 to 3 minutes until browned. Season with salt and garlic powder. Serve topped with fresh rosemary.

Spanish-style "tortilla De Patatas"

INGREDIENTS for Servings: 3

5 eggs, beaten	Salt and black pepper to taste
1 cup spinach, torn, rinsed	
	¼ tsp dried thyme
1 potato, chopped	1 tbsp olive oil
1 cup heavy cream	

DIRECTIONS and Cooking Time: 30 Minutes
In a bowl, mix eggs, heavy cream, and potato. Sprinkle with salt and black pepper, and stir to combine. Heat olive oil on Sauté and cook the spinach and thyme for 3 minutes, or until wilted. Remove the spinach from the pot. Stir in the spinach in the previously prepared mixture. Transfer all to an oven-safe dish, that fits in the Electric Pressure Cooker. Add 1 cup of water, insert the trivet, pour 1 cup of water, and place the oven-safe dish on top. Seal the lid and cook on High

Pressure for 20 minutes. Release the steam naturally, for 5 minutes.

Crushed Potatoes With Aioli

INGREDIENTS for Servings: 4

1 lb Russet potatoes, pierced	2 tbsp olive oil
Salt and black pepper to taste	4 tbsp mayonnaise
	1 tsp garlic paste
	1 tbsp lemon juice

DIRECTIONS and Cooking Time: 25 Minutes
Mix olive oil, salt, and pepper in a bowl. Add in the potatoes and toss to coat. Pour 1 cup of water in your Electric Pressure Cooker and fit in a trivet. Place the potatoes on the trivet and seal the lid. Select Manual and cook for 12 minutes on High. Once ready, perform a quick pressure release and unlock the lid. In a small bowl, combine mayonnaise, garlic paste, and lemon juice; mix well. Peel and crush the potatoes and transfer to a serving bowl. Serve with aioli.

Vegetarian Khoreshe Karafs (persian Celery Stew)

INGREDIENTS for Servings: 4

2 tablespoons unsalted butter	1 onion, chopped
2 garlic cloves, minced	2 tablespoons fresh mint, finely chopped
Sea salt and ground black pepper, to taste	2 tablespoons fresh cilantro, roughly chopped
1 teaspoon cayenne pepper	3 cups vegetable broth
1/2 teaspoon mustard seeds	1 Persian lime, prick a few holes
1 pound celery stalks, diced	2 cups basmati rice, steamed

DIRECTIONS and Cooking Time: 40 Minutes
Press the "Sauté" button and melt the butter. Once hot, cook the garlic and onions for about 3 minutes or until tender and fragrant. Stir in the spices, celery, herbs, broth, and Persian lime. Secure the lid. Choose the "Manual" mode and cook for 18 minutes at High pressure. Once cooking is complete, use a natural pressure release for 15 minutes; carefully remove the lid. Taste for seasoning and add more salt as needed. Serve with hot basmati rice and enjoy!

Kale And Sweet Potatoes With Tofu

INGREDIENTS for Servings: 4

1 tbsp. tamari sauce	8 oz. cubed tofu
2/3 cup vegetable broth	Salt and pepper, to taste
1 sweet potato, cubed	
2 cups chopped kale	

DIRECTIONS and Cooking Time: 6 Minutes

Add tofu in the Electric Pressure Cooker. Drizzle with half of the tamari and the broth. Cook for about 3 minutes on Sauté function. Add the rest of the ingredients. Lock the lid. Set the Electric Pressure Cooker to Manual mode, then set the timer for about 3 minutes at High Pressure. Once cooking is complete, do a quick pressure release. Carefully open the lid. Serve immediately!

Garlic & Leek Cannellini Beans

INGREDIENTS for Servings: 2-4

1 lb cannellini beans, soaked overnight	3 garlic cloves, whole
1 onion, peeled, chopped	1 tsp salt
	Topping:
2 large leeks, finely chopped	4 tbsp vegetable oil
	2 tbsp flour
1 tsp pepper	1 tbsp cayenne pepper

DIRECTIONS and Cooking Time: 45 Minutes
Add all ingredients, except for the topping ones, in the Electric Pressure Cooker. Press Manual/Pressure Cook and cook for 20 minutes on High. Meanwhile, heat 4 tbsp of oil in a skillet. Add flour and cayenne pepper. Stir-fry for 2 minutes and set aside. When you hear the cooker's end signal, do a quick release. Pour in the cayenne mixture and give it a good stir. Let it sit for 15 minutes before serving.

Maple Glazed Carrots

INGREDIENTS for Servings: 4-6

2/3 cup water	1 tbsp maple syrup
2 lbs carrots, sliced into ½ inch diagonal pieces	1 tbsp butter
	Salt and ground black pepper to taste
¼ cup raisins	

DIRECTIONS and Cooking Time: 40 Minutes
Add the water, carrots and raisins to the Electric Pressure Cooker. Secure the lid. Select the MANUAL setting and set the cooking time for 4 minutes at HIGH pressure. Once pressure cooking is complete, select CANCEL and use a Quick Release. Carefully unlock the lid. Transfer the carrots to a bowl. Carefully pour the water out of the pot and completely dry the pot before replacing it. Select SAUTÉ; add the butter and maple syrup. Return the carrots to the pot and stir well until fully coated with butter. Press the CANCEL key to stop the SAUTÉ function. Season with salt and pepper. Serve.

Hearty French Ratatouille

INGREDIENTS for Servings: 4

1 pound eggplant, sliced	1 cup vegetable broth
1 tablespoon sea salt	Sea salt and ground red pepper, to taste
1 pound zucchini,	1 teaspoon oregano

sliced 3 sweet peppers, seeded and sliced 2 onions, sliced 4 cloves garlic, pressed 1 pound tomatoes, pureed	1 teaspoon basil 1 teaspoon rosemary 4 tablespoons extra-virgin olive oil 4 tablespoons Pinot Noir

DIRECTIONS and Cooking Time: 40 Minutes

Toss the eggplant with 1 teaspoon of salt in a colander. Let it sit for 30 minutes; then squeeze out the excess liquid. Transfer the eggplant to the inner pot of your Electric Pressure Cooker. Add the other ingredients to the inner pot Secure the lid. Choose the "Manual" mode and cook for 6 minutes at High pressure. Once cooking is complete, use a quick pressure release; carefully remove the lid. Season to taste with salt and pepper and serve warm. Enjoy!

Monday Night Rice With Red Beans

INGREDIENTS for Servings: 4

1 cup red beans 2 tbsp vegetable oil ½ cup rice ½ tbsp cayenne pepper 1 ½ cup vegetable broth 1 onion, diced 1 garlic clove	1 red bell pepper, diced 1 stalk celery, diced 1 tbsp fresh thyme leaves Salt and black pepper to taste

DIRECTIONS and Cooking Time: 50 Minutes

Add beans and water to cover about 1-inch. Seal the lid and cook for 1 minute on High Pressure. Release the pressure quickly. Drain the beans and set aside. Rinse and pat dry the inner pot. Return inner pot to the cooker, add oil to the pot and press Sauté. Add onion to the oil and Sauté for 3 minutes until soft. Add celery and bell pepper and cook for 1 to 2 minutes until fragrant. Add garlic and cook for 30 seconds until soft. Add rice, transfer the beans back to the pot and top with broth. Stir black pepper, thyme, cayenne pepper, and salt into the mixture. Seal the lid and cook for 15 minutes on High Pressure. Release the pressure quickly. Season with more thyme, black pepper and salt.

BEEF & LAMB, PORK RECIPES

Burrito Beef

INGREDIENTS for Servings: 6

2 large scallions, chopped	½ tsp cumin
32-oz steak, cooked, boneless	4 tbsp green taco sauce
1 jalapeño pepper, minced	1 garlic clove, crushed
Salt and black pepper to taste	2 tbsp olive oil
2 tsp chili powder	½ cup green onions, chopped
	2 cups salsa verde

DIRECTIONS and Cooking Time: 56 Minutes
Set your IP to Sauté and heat the olive oil. Remove excess fat from steak and cook the meat on all sides for 5-6 minutes. In a bowl, mix jalapeño pepper, salsa verde, green onions, garlic, chili powder, cumin, salt, and pepper. Add mixture to the IP and stir well. Pour in 1 cup of water. Seal the lid, select Manual at High, and cook for 20 minutes. When ready, release the pressure naturally for 10 minutes. Remove the beef and shred it using two forks. Serve warm in burritos topped with green taco sauce.

Tagliatelle With Beef Sausage & Beans

INGREDIENTS for Servings: 6

1 lb beef sausages, chopped	2 tsp olive oil
1 lb dried tagliatelle pasta	1 cup scallions, chopped
½ cup dry white wine	1 (28-oz) can whole tomatoes
1 clove garlic, minced	¼ tsp crushed red pepper flakes
½ cups green peas, frozen	1 cup Grana Padano, grated
½ chipotle pepper, chopped	½ tsp dried basil
1 cup black beans, soaked	½ tsp dried oregano
2 yellow bell peppers, chopped	Salt and black pepper to taste
	Fresh parsley, for garnish

DIRECTIONS and Cooking Time: 30 Minutes
Heat oil in your IP on Sauté. Add scallions, bell peppers, and garlic and cook for 3 minutes. Stir in sausages and sear until lightly browned, for about 3-4 minutes. Add the remaining ingredients, except for parsley and Grana Padano cheese. Add 2 cups of water. Seal the lid, select Manual, and cook for 10 more minutes at High. Once ready, do a quick release. Stir in Grana Padano cheese until melted. Serve sprinkled with parsley.

Green Chili Pork With Pomodoro Sauce

INGREDIENTS for Servings: 6

1 ½ lb pork shoulder, cubed	¼ tsp green chili pepper
1 cup tomato puree	3 garlic cloves, minced
½ cups sour cream	½ tbsp cilantro
1 cup green onions, chopped	Salt and black pepper to taste
2 tsp butter, melted	

DIRECTIONS and Cooking Time: 35 Minutes
Melt butter on Sauté, and cook onions and garlic until soft, 2-3 minutes. Add the remaining ingredients, except for the sour cream. Seal the lid and cook for 25 minutes on Manual at High. Once cooking is over, do a quick pressure release. Stir in the sour cream until well incorporated. Serve.

Zucchini & Potato Beef Stew

INGREDIENTS for Servings: 4

1 lb beef round steak, sliced	2 zucchinis, sliced
1 clove garlic, minced	2 potatoes, chopped
2 tbsp olive oil	1 onion, chopped
1 cup buttermilk	2 cups vegetable broth
2 tbsp cornstarch	Salt and black pepper to taste
3 shallots, chopped	

DIRECTIONS and Cooking Time: 65 Minutes
Set your IP to Sauté and heat the olive oil. Add beef, shallots, garlic, potatoes, onion, salt, and pepper, and cook for 5-6 minutes, stirring often. Pour in broth, seal the lid, select Manual at High, and cook for 20 minutes. When ready, release the pressure quickly. Stir in zucchinis for 4-5 minutes on Sauté. In a bowl, mix together buttermilk and cornstarch. Add mixture to the pot and cook for a minute. Serve hot.

Thyme Creamy Beef Roast

INGREDIENTS for Servings: 6

1 ½ lb beef roast, cubed	1 tbsp garlic, minced
1 cup onion, diced	1 tbsp butter
14 oz canned mushroom soup	½ tsp chili powder
1 ½ cups buttermilk	½ tsp green chili powder
½ tbsp cumin	Salt and black pepper to taste
1 tbsp thyme	

DIRECTIONS and Cooking Time: 35 Minutes
Melt butter on Sauté in your IP and add in the onion and garlic. Cook until soft, about 3 minutes. Add beef and cook until browned, for about 5-6 minutes.

Combine the remaining ingredients in a bowl and pour this mixture over the beef. Pour in ½ cup of water. Seal the lid and cook for 25 minutes on Manual at High. Once done, do a quick release. Serve.

Jalapeño Ground Pork Stew

INGREDIENTS for Servings: 6

2 lb ground pork	3 tbsp butter
1 onion, diced	1 cup vegetable broth
1 can tomatoes, diced	1 tsp ground ginger
1 can green peas	2 tsp ground corriander
5 garlic cloves, crushed	Salt and black pepper to taste
1 jalapeño pepper, chopped	¼ tsp cayenne pepper

DIRECTIONS and Cooking Time: 60 Minutes
Melt butter on Sauté. Add onions and cook for 3 minutes until soft. Stir in the spices and garlic and cook for 2 more minutes. Add pork and cook until browned. Add broth, jalapeño, peas, and tomatoes. Seal the lid and cook for 30 minutes on Manual at High. Release pressure naturally for 10 minutes. Serve.

European Stew

INGREDIENTS for Servings: 6

1 lb pork loin, cubed	2 tsp dried marjoram
3 tbsp olive oil	1 tsp sugar
1 lb smoked sausage, sliced	2 tbsp red wine vinegar
3 ½ cups cooked beets, cubed	1 cup carrots, shredded
Salt and black pepper to taste	1 cup onions, sliced
1 cup sour cream	2 cups potatoes, shredded
2 tsp dill weed, chopped	4 cups cabbage, shredded

DIRECTIONS and Cooking Time: 55 Minutes
Set your IP to Sauté and heat the olive oil. Add all the ingredients, except for the sour cream, cabbage, potatoes, dill, and cook for 5-6 minutes, stirring often. Pour in 2 cups of water, potatoes, cabbage, and stir. Seal the lid, select Manual at High, and cook for 20 minutes. When ready, release the pressure naturally for 10 minutes. Serve warm and garnish each bowl with a dollop of sour cream and some dill weed.

Savory Baby Back Ribs

INGREDIENTS for Servings: 4

3 lb baby beef racks, cut individually	1 cup ale
2 tsp olive oil	12 oz barbecue sauce
Salt and black pepper to taste	½ tsp onion powder
	¼ tsp chipotle powder
	¼ tsp garlic powder

DIRECTIONS and Cooking Time: 50 Minutes

Mix all spices in a small bowl. Pour the mixture over meat; turn ribs to coat. Heat oil on Sauté, and sear the meat for 3 minutes per side, until browned. Insert the rack, arrange the ribs on top, and pour the ale over. Seal the lid, cook on Manual for 35 minutes at High. Do a quick release. Pour barbecue sauce over the ribs. Simmer for 5 minutes until sticky on Sauté.

Savory Beef Roast In Passion Fruit Gravy

INGREDIENTS for Servings: 8

3-4 lb beef roast	2 garlic cloves, minced
1 onion, peeled and quartered	1 tsp rosemary
3 ½ tbsp cornstarch	2 tbsp olive oil
1 ½ quarts passion fruit juice	Salt and black pepper to taste
1 cup beef broth	

DIRECTIONS and Cooking Time: 65 Minutes
Season the beef with salt, rosemary, and pepper. Warm oil and add pot roast; brown on all sides for 5-6 minutes on Sauté. Remove to a plate. Cook onion and garlic for 2 minutes. Pour broth to deglaze the bottom of the pot. Return the beef, seal the lid, select Manual, and cook for 45 minutes at High. Do a quick release, remove the roast to a plate. Whisk 4 tbsp of water and cornstarch and stir in the pot. Simmer until the gravy thickens. Slice the meat and drizzle the gravy over.

Spinach, Rice And Beef Sausage Stew

INGREDIENTS for Servings: 4

2 lb spinach, shredded	1 tsp fennel seeds, cooked
1 lb beef sausage, sliced	1 cup scallions, chopped
2 cloves garlic, minced	Salt and black pepper to taste
1 ½ cups canned tomatoes	½ cup fresh parsley, chopped
1 cup white rice, cooked	1 cup beef broth

DIRECTIONS and Cooking Time: 25 Minutes
In a mixing bowl, stir in spinach and fennel seeds. Take half of this mixture to make a bed at the bottom of the cooker. In another bowl, mix rice, sausage, parsley, scallions, garlic, salt, and pepper. Ladle half of this mixture over the spinach mixture and then top with another layer of the remaining spinach mixture. Finally, top with the remaining part of the meat mixture. In a large-sized bowl, whisk the tomatoes, and broth. Pour over the mixture. Select Manual seal the lid and cook for 15 minutes at High. Once the cooking is complete, do a quick pressure release. Serve in individual bowls, topped with parsley.

Greek-style Cooked Pulled Pork

INGREDIENTS for Servings: 4

2 tbsp Greek seasoning	2 lb pork tenderloin, fat trimmed
2 tbsp olive oil	2 tbsp fresh dill, chopped
1 jar sliced pepperoncini	

DIRECTIONS and Cooking Time: 46 Minutes
Sprinkle pork with the Greek seasoning. Heat the olive oil on Sauté in the IP and brown the pork on all sides for 5-6 minutes. Pour the jar of pepperoncini peppers and ½ cup of water over the pork. Seal the lid, select Manual at High, and cook for 20 minutes. When ready, release the pressure naturally for 10 minutes. Remove the pork and shred using two forks. Return the shredded pork to cooker and stir. Serve sprinkled with fresh dill.

Sage Pork Butt With Potatoes

INGREDIENTS for Servings: 4

1 lb pork butt, cubed	1 ½ tsp sage
1 lb potatoes, diced	1 ½ cups vegetable broth
2 tsp butter	Salt and black pepper to taste
¼ tsp thyme	
¼ tsp parsley	

DIRECTIONS and Cooking Time: 25 Minutes
Season pork with thyme, sage, parsley, salt, and pepper. Melt butter on Sauté. Add pork and brown, 6 minutes. Add the potatoes and pour in broth. Seal the lid and cook for 20 minutes on Manual at High. When ready, do a quick release, and serve hot.

Ground Pork Soup With Leeks & Carrots

INGREDIENTS for Servings: 6

1 lb ground pork	3 cups leeks, chopped
1 onion, diced	2 carrots, chopped
2 lb napa cabbage, chopped	1 tsp parsley
1 potato, diced	1 tbsp butter
6 button mushrooms, sliced	4 cups chicken broth
	Salt and black pepper to taste

DIRECTIONS and Cooking Time: 20 Minutes
Melt butter on Sauté and add the pork. Cook until browned, breaking it with a spatula. Once browned, add onion, leeks, and mushrooms, and cook for another 5 minutes. Season with salt and pepper. Pour in chicken broth and stir in the remaining ingredients. Seal the lid, cook on Manual for 6 minutes at High. Do a quick release. Ladle into Servings bowls to serve.

Butternut Squash Beef With Bok Choy

INGREDIENTS for Servings: 8

1 lb beef flank steak, sliced	2 tbsp olive oil
2 red onions, sliced	3 cloves garlic, minced
1 lb butternut squash, diced	2 carrots, diced
2 bell peppers, sliced	1 (6-oz) can tomato puree
1 cup bok choy, chopped	Salt and black pepper to taste

DIRECTIONS and Cooking Time: 50 Minutes
Heat the oil to Sauté and brown the meat on all sides, about 7-8 minutes; set aside. Lay vegetables at the bottom of the cooker and place the steak on top. In a bowl, mix in the remaining ingredients, and pour over the meat. Add in 2 cups of water. Seal the lid, select Manual, and cook for 30 minutes at High. Do a quick pressure release and serve.

Awesome Rutabaga And Pear Pork Loins

INGREDIENTS for Servings: 4

1 tbsp olive oil	1 celery stalk, diced
1 lb pork loin, cut into cubes	½ cup leeks, sliced
2 pears, peeled and chopped	1 ½ cups vegetable broth
2 rutabagas, chopped	½ tsp cumin
1 onion, diced	½ tsp thyme
1 tbsp parsley, chopped	Salt and black pepper to taste

DIRECTIONS and Cooking Time: 25 Minutes
Heat half of the olive oil on Sauté. Add pork and cook until browned on all sides. Remove to a plate. Add leeks, onions, celery, and drizzle with the remaining oil. Stir to combine and cook for 3 minutes. Add pork back to the cooker, pour the broth over, and stir in all the herbs and spices. Seal the lid, and cook on Manual at High for 10 minutes. After the beep, do a quick pressure release. Stir in rutabagas and pears. Seal the lid again and cook for 5 minutes on Manual at High. Do a quick pressure release, and serve right away.

Mediterranean Tomato Beef Soup

INGREDIENTS for Servings: 4

1 cup onions, diced	3 tsp garlic, minced
1 cup vegetable broth	¼ cup chopped basil
1 cup milk	1 tbsp sage
1 ½ cups ground beef	1 tbsp olive oil
30 oz canned tomatoes	Salt and black pepper to taste
1 carrot, chopped	

DIRECTIONS and Cooking Time: 35 Minutes
Heat oil on Sauté, add beef, and cook until browned on all sides. Add onions, carrot, and garlic, and saute for 2 minutes. Blend tomatoes and milk in a blender. Pour over the beef. Add the rest of the ingredients and stir to combine. Seal the lid, select Manual, and cook for 15 minutes at High. When done, do a quick release.

Mount-watering Beef Ribs With Shiitake

INGREDIENTS for Servings: 6

1 ½ lb beef ribs	1 cup carrots, chopped
2 cups Shiitake mushrooms	¼ cup sesame oil
1 onion, chopped	1 tsp garlic, minced
¼ cup ketchup	Salt and black pepper to taste
2 cups veggie stock	

DIRECTIONS and Cooking Time: 25 Minutes
Heat the oil on Sauté. Season the ribs with salt and pepper and brown them on all sides; set aside. Add the onion, garlic, carrots, and quartered mushrooms and cook for 5 minutes. Add the ribs back to the cooker and stir in the remaining ingredients. Seal the lid and cook for 35 minutes on Manual at High. When cooking is over, do a quick release. Serve hot.

Lamb Shanks In Port Wine

INGREDIENTS for Servings: 4

2 lb lamb shanks	1 tsp balsamic vinegar
1 tbsp olive oil	1 tsp sage
½ cup sweet white wine	1 tsp oregano
1 tbsp Tomato puree	½ tsp dried rosemary
1 carrot, chopped	1 tbsp butter
8 whole garlic cloves, peeled	Salt and black pepper to taste
½ cup chicken broth	

DIRECTIONS and Cooking Time: 50 Minutes
Season lamb shanks with salt and pepper. Warm oil and brown lamb on all sides, about 2-3 minutes on Sauté. Add garlic and cook until fragrant. Stir in the rest of the ingredients, except for butter and vinegar. Seal the lid, cook on Manual for 35 minutes at High. Do a quick pressure release. Remove lamb shanks and let the sauce boil for 5 minutes on Sauté. Stir in vinegar and butter. Serve, with the gravy drizzle over shanks.

Dinner Ribs With Beets And Potatoes

INGREDIENTS for Servings: 6

1 ½ cups beef broth	2 lb short ribs, excess fat trimmed
½ lb small potatoes	
3 tsp butter	½ lb beets, thinly sliced
2 red onions, chopped	

1 tbsp thyme	Salt and black pepper to taste
1 (14.5-ounce) can tomatoes	
2 sprigs rosemary	2 cloves garlic, minced

DIRECTIONS and Cooking Time: 55 Minutes
Rub the ribs with salt and black pepper. Heat the oil on Sauté and sear the spare ribs on all sides. Set aside. Add the beets, garlic, and onion; stir-fry for another 4-5 minutes. Return the ribs to the pressure cooker and stir in the remaining ingredients. Pour in ½ cup of water. Seal the lid and cook for 45 minutes on Manual at High. Once cooking is complete, perform a quick pressure release and remove the lid. Serve immediately.

Pork Shoulder Roast With Noodles

INGREDIENTS for Servings: 6

3 lb boneless pork shoulder	1 cup onion, chopped
	3 tbsp cornstarch
3 tbsp olive oil	1 cup chicken broth
2 tbsp oregano	Salt and black pepper to taste
6 cups cooked noodles	

DIRECTIONS and Cooking Time: 51 Minutes
Heat the olive oil on Sauté and brown the pork on all sides for 5-6 minutes. Set aside. Add in the onion and cook for 3 minutes until soften. Return the pork, pour in the broth, and 1 cup of water. Season with salt, pepper, and oregano. Seal the lid, select Manual at High, and cook for 20 minutes. When ready, release the pressure naturally for 10 minutes. Remove the pork from pot and shred it with two forks. In a small bowl, mix the cornstarch with a cup of the cooking liquid and pour in the IP. Cook on Sauté for 2-3 minutes until thickened. Return in the shredded pork and stir. Serve over a bed of noodles.

Sliced Beef Steak With Carrots

INGREDIENTS for Servings: 4

2 lb beef eye round steak, sliced	1 bay leaf
	½ cup bell peppers, chopped
2 tbsp olive oil	
Salt and black pepper to taste	½ cup carrots, sliced
	½ cup onions, sliced
1 can (14-oz) tomatoes, diced	1 cup celery, sliced
	1 ½ cups beef broth
2 garlic cloves, diced	1 tbsp liquid smoke
	Chopped green onions

DIRECTIONS and Cooking Time: 1 Hour And 19 Minutes
Set your IP to Sauté and heat olive oil. Add onions, bell peppers, celery, garlic, carrots, salt, and pepper and cook for 5 minutes, stirring often. Add in beef and brown for 3-4 minutes on both sides. Pour in broth, bay leaf, liquid smoke, and tomatoes. Seal the lid, select Manual at High, and cook for 40 minutes. When

ready, release the pressure quickly. Discard the bay leaf. Serve topped with freshly chopped green onions.

Sweet Shredded Pork

INGREDIENTS for Servings: 6

2 lb pork shoulder	2 tbsp maple syrup
Salt and black pepper to taste	1 large sweet onion, chopped
1 tsp allspice	3 peaches, pitted and sliced
1 tsp garlic powder	1 cup vegetable broth
1 tbsp fresh ginger, minced	

DIRECTIONS and Cooking Time: 50 Minutes
Pour broth and add pork to the IP. Add peaches, maple syrup, onion, ginger, garlic powder, salt, pepper, and allspice, and broth. Seal the lid, select Manual at High, and cook for 30 minutes. When ready, release the pressure naturally for 10 minutes. Remove the pork and shred it using two forks, then stir back to cooker.

Mom's Rump Roast With Potatoes

INGREDIENTS for Servings: 6

3 lb rump roast	2 cups beef broth
6 Yukon gold, quartered	1 tbsp butter
1 onion, diced	1 carrot, chopped
1 tsp sage	1 tbsp butter
1 celery stalk, chopped	2 garlic cloves, minced
1 ½ tbsp Dijon mustard	Salt and black pepper to taste

DIRECTIONS and Cooking Time: 65 Minutes
Heat the oil on Sauté. Add onion and celery, and cook for 4 minutes until soft. Brush the mustard over the beef and season with salt and pepper. Place in the pot and sear on all sides for 5 minutes. Stir in the remaining ingredients and seal the lid. Cook for 45 minutes on Manual at High. Do a natural release for 10 minutes.

Chili Beef Brisket With Chives

INGREDIENTS for Servings: 6

2 ½ lb beef brisket	1 cup vegetable broth
1 tbsp green chili powder	1 tbsp butter
½ cup tomato puree	1 onion, sliced
½ cup salsa	2 garlic cloves, minced
1 tbsp chives, chopped	Salt and black pepper to taste

DIRECTIONS and Cooking Time: 60 Minutes
Season the beef with green chili powder. Coat the inner pot with cooking spray, press Sauté and brown beef on all sides, about 6 minutes. Add onion and cook for 2 more minutes until soft. Stir in the remaining ingredients. Seal the lid and cook for 35 minutes on Manual at High. Do a quick pressure release and serve.

Sage Pork Ribs In Pecan Sauce

INGREDIENTS for Servings: 4

¼ cup roasted pecans, chopped	1 lb pork ribs
4 garlic cloves, minced	3 tbsp butter
1 ½ cups vegetable broth	½ tsp red pepper flakes
2 tbsp apple cider vinegar	1 tsp sage
	1 tsp oregano
	Salt and black pepper to taste

DIRECTIONS and Cooking Time: 30 Minutes
Melt butter on Sauté. Season the ribs with salt, pepper, sage, and red pepper flakes. Place them in the pressure cooker and brown for about 5 minutes. Stir in the remaining ingredients. Seal the lid. Cook for 20 minutes on Manual at High. Release the pressure quickly. Serve drizzled with the sauce.

Quick Pork Chops With Cabbage

INGREDIENTS for Servings: 4

4 pork chops	1 tbsp olive oil
½ lb cabbage	1 cup celery stalk, chopped
¼ cup sparkling wine	1 tbsp thyme
1 ½ cups vegetable stock	Salt and black pepper to taste
2 shallots, chopped	

DIRECTIONS and Cooking Time: 35 Minutes
Heat olive oil on Sauté. Add the pork chops and cook until browned on all sides. Stir in the remaining ingredients. Seal the lid and cook for 25 minutes on Manual at High. Release the pressure quickly.

Lamb With Green Onions

INGREDIENTS for Servings: 4

Salt and black pepper to taste	1 lb lamb chops
1 cup tomatoes, chopped	2 cups chicken stock
4 cups green onions, chopped	1 tsp paprika
2 garlic cloves, minced	2 tbsp mint, chopped
	2 tbsp parsley, chopped
	3 tbsp olive oil

DIRECTIONS and Cooking Time: 45 Minutes
Select Sauté on your IP and heat olive oil. Cook green onions and garlic for 4 minutes until soft. Add in lamb and cook for 6 minutes on both sides. Season with salt, pepper, add paprika and stir. Pour in chicken stock, tomatoes, and mint. Seal the lid, select Manual, and cook for 15 minutes at High. Once cooking is over, do a quick pressure release. Ladle into individual plates and serve topped with fresh parsley.

Tender Bbq Ribs

INGREDIENTS for Servings: 6

1 (3 lb) rack pork spare ribs	1 cup vegetable broth
5 tbsp chili sauce	1 tsp dried mustard
Salt and black pepper to taste	1 cup BBQ sauce
	2 tbsp balsamic vinegar

DIRECTIONS and Cooking Time: 55 Minutes
Remove the membrane from the ribs. Cut the rack of ribs into portions. Put them in the IP. Combine the remaining ingredients in a bowl and pour over the pork. Seal the lid, select Manual at High, and cook for 30 minutes. When ready, release the pressure naturally for 10 minutes. Serve hot topped with cooking sauce.

Pork Ribs With Tomato And Carrots

INGREDIENTS for Servings: 4

1 ½ cups tomato sauce	½ cup carrots, thinly sliced
1 tbsp garlic, minced	1 lb cut pork spare ribs
Salt and black pepper to taste	2 tbsp olive oil
½ tsp dried sage	
1 ¼ cups green onions	

DIRECTIONS and Cooking Time: 35 Minutes
Heat oil in your IP on Sauté and brown the ribs for 7-8 minutes. Pour in 1 ½ cups of water and tomato sauce. Add the remaining ingredients. Seal the lid and cook for 30 minutes on Manual at High. Once ready, do a quick pressure release and serve.

Pork Chops With Sage

INGREDIENTS for Servings: 4

4 loin chops, boneless	½ cup chicken broth
2 tbsp Dijon mustard	½ cup dry white wine
1 tbsp cornstarch	¼ cup onion, chopped
2 tbsp lemon juice	Salt and black pepper to taste
2 tbsp honey	2 tbsp sage, chopped
2 tbsp water	

DIRECTIONS and Cooking Time: 43 Minutes
Pour wine, onion, broth, and pork chops into the IP. Seal the lid, select Manual at High, and cook for 10 minutes. When ready, release the pressure naturally for 10 minutes. Transfer the pork to a platter and keep warm. Set your IP to Sauté and add in the honey, water, mustard, lemon juice, and cornstarch and stir to combine. Cook for about 2-3 minutes while stirring often, on Sauté. Serve warm sprinkled with sage.

Pork With Prune Sauce

INGREDIENTS for Servings: 4

1 ¼ lb pork tenderloin	½ cup pear juice
1 chopped celery stalk	¼ cup onions, chopped
2 cups pears, chopped	Salt and black pepper to taste
1 cup prunes, pitted	2 tbsp olive oil

DIRECTIONS and Cooking Time: 60 Minutes
Heat oil in your IP on Sauté and cook the onions and celery for 5 minutes until softened. Season pork with salt and pepper, and add to the cooker. Brown for 2-3 minutes per side. Top with pears and prunes, and pour in ½ cup of water and pear juice. Seal the lid and cook on Manual for 35 minutes at High. Do a quick pressure release. Slice the pork and arrange on a platter. Spoon the sauce over the pork slices to serve.

Autumn Beef Stew

INGREDIENTS for Servings: 6

3 ½ lb stew beef meat, cubed	1 rutabaga, chopped
½ cup ghee	Salt and black pepper to taste
2 tbsp ground cumin	2 cinnamon sticks
1 cup beef broth	2 bay leaves
1 can (14-oz) tomatoes	1 tsp coriander seeds, ground
4 cloves garlic, minced	1 tbsp paprika
1 onion, chopped	Chopped parsley for garnish
5 zucchinis, diced	

DIRECTIONS and Cooking Time: 47 Minutes
Set your IP to Sauté and melt the ghee. Cook the garlic and onion for 3-4 minutes. Add in the beef and cook for 5-6 minutes until brown. Stir in the tomatoes, broth, cumin, coriander, paprika, and cook for 5 minutes. Add in the bay leaves, rutabaga, and cinnamon sticks. Seal the lid, select Manual at High, and cook for 18 minutes. When ready, do a quick release. Add the zucchinis, set to Sauté and cook for an additional 5 minutes. Season with salt and pepper. Serve hot, garnished with parsley.

Spiced Beef Brisket & Pancetta Stew

INGREDIENTS for Servings: 4

1 ½ lb beef brisket, cubed	2 tsp chipotle powder
2 slices pancetta, diced	2 cups green onion, chopped
2 garlic cloves, smashed	2 tbsp red wine
2 red bell peppers, minced	2 cups beef stock
3 potatoes, peeled and diced	2 tomatoes, finely chopped
1 tbsp butter, softened	1 tsp chili pepper, minced
	Salt and black pepper to taste

DIRECTIONS and Cooking Time: 40 Minutes
Melt butter on Sauté. Place the pancetta and beef, and brown them for 3 minutes, stirring occasionally. Add in the remaining ingredients. Seal the lid, and cook for

30 minutes on Manual at High. Once cooking is over, do a quick pressure release. Serve.

Beef And Sauerkraut Dinner

INGREDIENTS for Servings: 6

1 ½ lb ground beef	3 cups sauerkraut
10 oz canned tomato soup	1 tbsp butter
	1 tsp mustard powder
½ cup vegetable broth	Salt and black pepper to taste
1 cup green onions, chopped	

DIRECTIONS and Cooking Time: 30 Minutes
Melt butter on Sauté in your IP. Add green onions and cook for a few minutes until soft. Add beef and brown for a few minutes. Stir in sauerkraut, broth, soup and mustard powder and season with salt and pepper. Seal the lid and cook for 20 minutes on Manual at High. When ready, do a quick pressure release. Serve.

Beef Paprikash

INGREDIENTS for Servings: 6

3 lb beef stew meat, cubed	1 tbsp sweet paprika
	2 bay leaves
2 cups red onions, chopped	3 tbsp old bay seasoning
3 tbsp olive oil	3 red bell peppers, chopped
1 cup sour cream	
1 tbsp chopped chives	Salt and black pepper to taste
3 tbsp tomato paste	

DIRECTIONS and Cooking Time: 67 Minutes
Set your IP to Sauté and heat the olive oil. Add the onions, bell peppers, and beef meat, and cook for 4-5 minutes. Stir in paprika, tomato paste, and old bay seasoning. Pour in the 1 cup of water and bay leaves. Seal the lid, select Manual at High, and cook for 25 minutes. When ready, release the pressure naturally for 10 minutes. Remove the bay leaves and season to taste with salt and pepper. Stir in sour cream and cook for 2 more minutes on Sauté. Serve warm with chives.

Pancetta & Cheese Rigatoni

INGREDIENTS for Servings: 6

1 ½ box penne pasta	1 cup yellow onions, chopped
6 slices pancetta, crumbled	3 garlic cloves, finely minced
½ cup Parmesan, grated	Salt and black pepper to taste
1 cup cottage cheese	
3 tsp olive oil	

DIRECTIONS and Cooking Time: 25 Minutes
Add pasta, 4 cups of water, salt, and black pepper in your IP. Seal the lid, select Manual, and cook for 4 minutes at High. Once ready, do a quick pressure release. Drain and set aside. Select Sauté and heat olive oil. Cook onions, garlic, and pancetta for 3 minutes. Return the pasta and stir in cottage cheese. Serve topped with grated Parmesan cheese.

Saucy Beef Short Ribs

INGREDIENTS for Servings: 4

2 lb beef short ribs, cut into pieces	½ cup red wine
	3 tbsp oil
Salt and black pepper to taste	½ tbsp tomato puree
	2 carrots, sliced
1 onion, chopped	

DIRECTIONS and Cooking Time: 60 Minutes
Rub ribs with salt and pepper. Heat oil on Sauté, and brown ribs on all sides, 8 minutes. Remove to a plate. Add onion and cook for 3 minutes. Pour in wine and tomato puree; deglaze by scraping any browned bits from the bottom of the pot. Cook for 2 minutes until wine has reduced slightly. Return ribs to the pot and add carrots. Pour 2 cups water. Seal the lid, select Manual at High, and cook for 30 minutes. When ready, let pressure release naturally for 10 minutes. Transfer ribs to a baking sheet and take under a broiler for 5 minutes until crispy. Take the remaining ingredients from the pot, to a food processor and blend until smooth. Serve the ribs topped with the blended sauce.

Lamb Cacciatore

INGREDIENTS for Servings: 4

1 lb lamb chops	1 onion, chopped
Salt and black pepper to taste	1 cup dry white wine
	2 cans (14-oz) tomatoes
3 tbsp olive oil	
¼ red bell pepper, sliced	1 cup chicken stock
2 cups mushrooms, sliced	2 tbsp black olives, pitted
	1 cup spinach, chopped
2 garlic cloves, minced	
	½ tsp dried oregano

DIRECTIONS and Cooking Time: 45 Minutes
Season lamb with salt and pepper. Select Sauté and heat oil. Cook lamb for 8 minutes; set aside. Add in bell pepper, onion, and mushrooms. Cook for 7 minutes. Pour in wine and garlic and cook for 2 minutes. Mix in tomatoes, stock, olives, spinach, oregano, and the lamb, along with any juices, Seal the lid, select Manual, and cook for 30 minutes at High. When done, do a natural pressure release for about 10 minutes. Serve.

Tasty Beef With Carrot-onion Gravy

INGREDIENTS for Servings: 4

4 round steaks	1 carrot, chopped
2 onions, sliced	½ tsp red pepper flakes
1 ½ cups beef broth	
1 tsp garlic, minced	¼ cup whipping

1 tbsp dried thyme ½ tsp rosemary 1 tbsp oil	cream 2 tbsp flour Salt and black pepper to taste

DIRECTIONS and Cooking Time: 40 Minutes
Heat oil on Sauté. Add beef and brown on all sides for 6 minutes. Remove to a plate. Sauté onions, carrot, and garlic for 2 minutes until fragrant. Return the steaks to the pressure cooker. Stir in the salt, black pepper, pepper flakes, rosemary, thyme, and pour in broth. Seal the lid and cook for 25 minutes on Manual at High. When ready, do a quick pressure release, and stir in the flour and whipping cream. Cook for 3 more minutes until thickened, lid off, on Sauté. Serve immediately.

Sunday Beef Roast With Garam Masala

INGREDIENTS for Servings: 8

3 lb beef roast ½ cup tomato puree ½ cup red wine 2 tsp soy sauce 1 tbsp brown sugar 1 tbsp balsamic vinegar 2 tbsp onions, minced 2 tsp mustard powder	1 tsp cayenne pepper powder 1 tsp garlic, minced ¼ tsp Garam masala ½ tsp cinnamon ground 1 tbsp rosemary Salt and black pepper to taste

DIRECTIONS and Cooking Time: 60 Minutes
Place beef in your IP. Whisk the remaining ingredients in a bowl. Pour this mixture over the beef with 1 cup of water. Seal the lid and cook for 40 minutes on Manual at High. When ready, release pressure quickly. Serve.

Curried Pork Stew With Peas

INGREDIENTS for Servings: 6

2 lb lean pork loin, cubed 1 ½ cups onions, chopped 1 ½ cups chicken broth Salt and black pepper to taste	1 ½ tsp curry powder 2 bay leaves 2 tbsp olive oil Chopped chives 1 cup frozen peas, thawed 1 large tomato, chopped

DIRECTIONS and Cooking Time: 35 Minutes
Set your IP to Sauté and heat olive oil. Add onions, pork, curry powder, salt, and pepper, and cook for 5-6 minutes, stirring often. Pour in broth, tomato, and bay leaves. Seal the lid, select Manual at High, and cook for 14 minutes. When ready, do a quick release. Remove and discard the bay leaves. Stir in the peas and cook for 5 minutes on Sauté. Serve topped with chives.

Veggie Beef Steak With Beer Sauce

INGREDIENTS for Servings: 6

2 lb beef steak, cut into 6 or 8 equal pieces 1 sweet onion, chopped 1 cup celery, chopped 1 lb sweet potatoes, diced 2 parsnips, chopped 3 garlic cloves, minced	2 bell peppers, chopped 1 ½ cups tomato puree 1 cup beer 1 tbsp sage 1 chicken bouillon cube Salt and black pepper to taste 1 tbsp olive oil

DIRECTIONS and Cooking Time: 50 Minutes
Heat oil on Sauté and sear the meat for a few minutes; set aside. Press Cancel. Arrange the veggies in the pressure cooker and top with the steak. In a bowl, whisk together bouillon cube, beer, sage, and tomato puree. Pour over the steaks. Season with salt and pepper, and seal the lid. Cook for 30 minutes on Manual at High. Quick-release the pressure, and serve.

Pork Shoulder In Bbq Sauce

INGREDIENTS for Servings: 8

4 lb pork shoulder 1 tbsp onion powder 1 tbsp garlic powder Salt and black pepper to taste 1 tbsp sweet chili powder	2 cups vegetable stock For BBQ sauce: 6 dates, soaked ¼ cup tomato puree ½ cup coconut aminos

DIRECTIONS and Cooking Time: 80 Minutes
In a small bowl, combine onion powder, garlic powder, pepper, salt, and sweet chili powder. Rub the mixture onto the pork. Place the pork in your pressure cooker. Pour the stock around the meat, not over it, and then seal the lid. Select Manual and set the timer to 60 minutes at High. Place all sauce ingredients in a food processor and pulse until smooth. Release the pressure quickly. Grab two forks and shred the meat inside the pot. Pour the sauce over and stir to combine. Serve.

Cilantro Vegetable Beef Soup

INGREDIENTS for Servings: 6

1 lb beef stew meat, cubed 1 ½ Russet potatoes, diced 2 tomatoes, chopped 1 cup stalk celery, chopped 1 cup carrots, diced 1 cup turnips, diced	1 cup green onions, chopped 5 cups beef broth Salt and black pepper to taste 1 tsp sage ½ cup fresh cilantro, chopped

DIRECTIONS and Cooking Time: 45 Minutes
In your pressure cooker, mix in all ingredients, except for the cilantro. Select Manual and adjust the cooking time for to 30 minutes at High. Seal the lid and switch the pressure release valve to close. Once the cooking is over, allow for natural pressure release for 10 minutes. Open the lid and stir in the cilantro. Serve warm.

Picante Beef Stew With Barley
INGREDIENTS for Servings: 8

2 lb beef stew meat, cubed	2 cups barley, rinsed
2 tbsp cayenne pepper	1 tsp oregano
2 tsp soy sauce	½ tsp red pepper flakes, crushed
2 (14.5 oz) cans tomatoes	Salt and black pepper to taste

DIRECTIONS and Cooking Time: 45 Minutes
Select Sauté and brown the beef for 5 minutes, stirring occasionally. Add the rest of the ingredients, 4 cups of water, and stir. Seal the lid, press Manual, and cook for 30 minutes at High. When ready, do a quick release. Adjust the seasoning. Fluff barley with a fork to serve.

Lamb & Mushroom Ragout
INGREDIENTS for Servings: 4

2 lb lamb, bone-in	1 yellow onion, chopped
2 tbsp butter	2 carrots, sliced
4 tomatoes, chopped	1 tsp rosemary
2 tbsp tomato puree	Salt and black pepper to taste
1 cup mushrooms, sliced	Fresh mint leaves, chopped
2 cloves garlic, minced	

DIRECTIONS and Cooking Time: 45 Minutes
Season lamb with salt and pepper. Melt butter on Sauté, add lamb and cook until browned on all sides, about 10 minutes. Stir in tomatoes, tomato puree, mushrooms, garlic, onion, carrots, and rosemary. Cover with 2 cups of water. Seal the lid, press Manual, and cook for 45 minutes at High. When ready, do a natural pressure release for 10 minutes. Discard bones from lamb and using two forks, shred it. Bring the lamb back to the pot and stir. Serve topped with chopped mint.

Pork & Mushrooms
INGREDIENTS for Servings: 4

1 lb lean pork loin, cubed	1 cup shallots, chopped
2 tbsp olive oil	1 cup mushrooms, sliced
1 ½ cups chicken broth	Salt and black pepper to taste
1 clove garlic, minced	16 oz egg noodles, cooked
1 cup sour cream	

DIRECTIONS and Cooking Time: 35 Minutes
Set your IP to Sauté and heat olive oil. Add shallots, garlic, mushrooms, and pork, and cook for 4-5 minutes, stirring often. Pour in broth and season with salt and pepper. Seal the lid, select Manual at High, and cook for 20 minutes. When ready, release the pressure naturally for 10 minutes. Stir in sour cream. Serve hot over a warm bed of cooked egg noodles.

Cuban Style Pork
INGREDIENTS for Servings: 4

2 lb pork shoulder roast	1 bay leaf
1 tsp oregano	4 garlic cloves, minced
2 tbsp olive oil	¼ tsp red pepper flakes
1 sweet onion, chopped	½ cup orange juice
Black pepper and salt to taste	Chopped chives, for garnish

DIRECTIONS and Cooking Time: 65 Minutes
Mix all the ingredients together in a bowl, except for the pork. Make cuts into the pork and place it inside the pot. Pour the mixture into the cuts on the meat. Add in 2 cups of water. Seal the lid, select Manual at High, and cook for 40 minutes. When ready, release the pressure naturally for 10 minutes. Remove and discard the bay leaf. Slice the meat. Serve hot, topped with cooking juices and sprinkled with freshly chopped chives.

Sweet & Sour Pork
INGREDIENTS for Servings: 4

1 ½ lb pork tenderloin, cubed	¼ cup soy sauce
1 whole hot red chili pepper	1 green bell pepper, diced
½ cup chicken broth	1 red bell pepper, diced
2 cloves garlic, sliced	2 tbsp potato flour
1 white onion, chopped	¼ cup fresh orange juice
1 cup pineapples, diced	½ tsp ground ginger
	1 tbsp raw honey
	3 tbsp tomato paste

DIRECTIONS and Cooking Time: 28 Minutes
Add all ingredients to the IP, except for the pineapples, bell peppers, potato flour and orange juice. Pour in 1 cup of water. Seal the lid, select Manual at High, and cook for 10 minutes. Perform a natural pressure release for 5 minutes. Mix the potato flour and orange juice in a mixing bowl to obtain a smooth paste. Add the paste to the cooker, along with the pineapple and peppers. Cook for 2-3 minutes on Sauté. Remove and discard the chili pepper and serve.

Herbed Veggie Beef Rib Eye

INGREDIENTS for Servings: 4

2 beef ribeye steaks	2 tsp flour
1 cup sweet onions, chopped	2 oz Italian salad dressing mix
¼ cup tomato sauce	½ tsp celery seeds
1 tsp garlic, minced	Salt and black pepper to taste
½ lb carrots, chopped	½ tsp cayenne pepper
2 ½ cups beef broth	
2 tsp butter	

DIRECTIONS and Cooking Time: 50 Minutes
Melt butter on Sauté. Add in meat and brown for 4 minutes, turning occasionally. Add the rest of the ingredients, except for the flour, and stir. Seal the lid and cook on Manual for 35 minutes at High. Once ready, do a quick pressure release. In a bowl, whisk together the flour with ¼ cup of cooking liquid. Add to the pot. Stir until everything is well combined. Serve.

Pineapple & Soda-glazed Ham

INGREDIENTS for Servings: 6

4 lb picnic ham	1 (15 ¼-oz) can pineapple rings with juice
1 can cola-flavored soda	

DIRECTIONS and Cooking Time: 33 Minutes
Add the ham to the IP with the fattier side facing downwards. Place the pineapple rings over the ham, attach them with toothpicks. Pour soda and pineapple juice, all over the ham. Seal the lid, select Manual at High, and cook for 8 minutes. When ready, release the pressure naturally for 5 minutes. Serve hot or cold.

Juicy Chorizo Sausage With Tater Tots

INGREDIENTS for Servings: 6

1 lb chorizo sausage, sliced	1 lb tater tots
1 lb cauliflower florets	10 oz canned cauliflower soup
10 oz canned mushroom soup	10 oz evaporated milk
	Salt and black pepper to taste

DIRECTIONS and Cooking Time: 25 Minutes
Place roughly ¼ of the sausage slices in your pressure cooker. In a bowl, whisk together the soups and milk. Pour some of this mixture over the sausages. Top the sausage slices with ¼ of the cauliflower florets followed by ¼ of the tater tots. Pour some of the soup mixtures again. Repeat the layers until you use up all ingredients. Seal the lid, and cook on Manual for 10 minutes at High. When ready, do a quick release.

Cheese Beef Taco Pie

INGREDIENTS for Servings: 4

1 package corn tortillas	12 oz Colby cheese
1 packet of taco seasoning	¼ cup refried beans
1 lb ground beef	Salt and black pepper to taste

DIRECTIONS and Cooking Time: 20 Minutes
Combine meat with the seasoning. Pour 1 cup of water in your IP and insert a trivet. Place 1 tortilla at the bottom of a baking pan and lay on the trivet. Top with beans, beef, and cheese. Top with another tortilla. Repeat until you've use up all ingredients. The final layer should be a tortilla. Seal the lid, and cook for 12 minutes on Manual at High. When ready, do a quick pressure release. Remove the pan and serve.

Pork Soup With Red Wine

INGREDIENTS for Servings: 4

4 cups chicken stock	2 bay leaves
2 tbsp olive oil	½ cup dry red wine
1 ½ tsp dried thyme	1 (14-oz) can tomato sauce
2 celery sticks, sliced	1 pound pork loin, cubed
½ cup carrots, sliced	
1 cup onions, chopped	6 oz Canadian bacon, diced
1 clove garlic, minced	
2 cups red potatoes, cubed	Salt and black pepper to taste

DIRECTIONS and Cooking Time: 55 Minutes
Set your IP to Sauté and heat olive oil. Add the onions, garlic, celery, carrots, bacon, and pork and cook for 4-5 minutes, stirring often. Pour in the stock, tomato sauce, bay leaves, thyme, potatoes, and red wine, and season with salt and pepper. Seal the lid, select Manual at High, and cook for 20 minutes. When ready, release the pressure naturally for 10 minutes. Discard the bay leaves. Adjust the seasoning and serve hot.

Pork Infused With Orange Juice

INGREDIENTS for Servings: 5

1 orange, cut in half	¼ tsp red pepper
2 tsp oregano	2 tbsp olive oil
1 sweet onion, chopped	3 garlic cloves, grated
½ tsp chili powder	1 jalapeño pepper, minced
Salt and black pepper to taste	Green onions for garnish
2 lb boneless pork shoulder	

DIRECTIONS and Cooking Time: 50 Minutes
In a bowl, mix spices and olive oil, then rub mixture onto pork. Add the remaining ingredients along with the pork to the IP, and pour in 1 cup of water. Seal the

lid, select Manual at High, and cook for 30 minutes. When ready, release the pressure naturally for 10 minutes. Serve hot, topped with chopped green onions.

Papaya Short Ribs

INGREDIENTS for Servings: 6

1 lb short ribs, cut into pieces	1 cup onions, sliced
18 oz canned papaya, undrained	½ tsp garlic, minced
	½ cup tomato puree
½ tsp parsley, chopped	3 tsp olive oil
	½ cup soy sauce
Salt and black pepper to taste	2 tbsp apple cider vinegar
1-inch piece ginger, grated	¼ cup prepared arrowroot slurry

DIRECTIONS and Cooking Time: 30 Minutes
On Sauté, heat oil and cook onions until tender, about 4 minutes. Stir in the remaining ingredients, except for arrowroot. Seal the lid, press Manual, and cook for 20 minutes at High. Once ready, do a quick release. Stir in the slurry and cook on Sauté until the sauce thickens.

Pork Meatballs With Sour Mushroom Sauce

INGREDIENTS for Servings: 4

Pork Meatballs:	Mushroom sauce:
1 ½ lbs ground pork	1 cup chicken broth
1 tsp salt	Salt and black pepper to taste
½ cup breadcrumbs	16 oz fettuccine, cooked
1 egg	
1 clove garlic, minced	3 tbsp cornstarch
¼ cup chopped green onions	1 cup sour cream
¼ tsp black pepper	8 oz mushrooms, sliced

DIRECTIONS and Cooking Time: 35 Minutes
In a bowl, mix all meatball ingredients, and shape into 8 meatballs; set aside. Arrange ¾ of the mushrooms at the bottom of the IP, top with meatballs, then the remaining mushrooms, and finally pour the broth over. Seal the lid, select Manual at High, and cook for 11 minutes. When ready, release the pressure naturally for 10 minutes. Remove the meatballs. Add in sour cream and cornstarch and stir for a few minutes on Sauté. Season to taste, and serve meatballs with the sauce.

Hungarian Bean Soup

INGREDIENTS for Servings: 5

1 lb beef round steak, cubed	Salt and black pepper to taste
3 tbsp olive oil	½ cup sour cream
5 cups beef broth	1 tsp dried thyme
1 cup red bell peppers, sliced	leaves
1 cup carrots, chopped	2 tsp crushed caraway seeds
3 cups cabbage, sliced	1 tbsp garlic, minced
1 cup onions, chopped	1 tbsp paprika
	1 (14-oz) can white beans

DIRECTIONS and Cooking Time: 46 Minutes
Set your IP to Sauté and heat the olive oil. Add the beef, onions, paprika, garlic, caraway seeds, thyme, carrots, cabbage, red bell peppers, salt, and pepper, and cook for 5-6 minutes. Pour in the broth and white beans. Seal the lid, select Manual at High, and cook for 15 minutes. When ready, do a quick release. Serve topped with a dollop of sour cream on each bowl.

Beef Roast With Onions

INGREDIENTS for Servings: 8

3 lb beef roast	1 tsp garlic, minced
2 large sweet onions, sliced	2 tbsp Worcestershire sauce
1 envelope onion mix	1 tbsp olive oil
1 cup beef broth	Salt and black pepper to taste
1 cup canned tomatoes	
1 tbsp cilantro	

DIRECTIONS and Cooking Time: 60 Minutes
Warm oil on Sauté. Season beef with salt and pepper, and sear on all sides. Transfer to a plate. Add onions, and cook for 3 minutes. Stir in garlic and cook for 1 minute. Add beef and stir in the remaining ingredients. Seal the lid and cook for 40 minutes on Manual at High. Release pressure naturally for 10 minutes. Serve.

Pork Chops With Broccoli

INGREDIENTS for Servings: 4

1 lb pork chops	1 tbsp arrowroot
1 cup onions, sliced	1 tsp garlic, minced
1 cup carrots, sliced	1 cup chicken stock
1 tbsp butter	½ tsp dried thyme
2 cups broccoli florets	Salt and black pepper to taste

DIRECTIONS and Cooking Time: 35 Minutes
Melt butter on Sauté. Add pork chops, and cook on all sides until golden. Transfer to a plate. Add onions, and cook for 3 minutes, then add garlic. Sauté for one minute. Return the pork chops to the pot and pour the broth over. Seal the lid and cook on Manual at High for 15 minutes. When done, do a quick pressure release. Stir in carrots and broccoli florets. Seal the lid again, and cook for 3 minutes on Manual at High. Do a quick pressure release. Transfer the chops and veggies to a Servings platter. Whisk the arrowroot into the pot and cook on Sauté until it thickens. Pour the sauce over the chops and veggies. Serve immediately.

Well-made Cheesy Meatballs

INGREDIENTS for Servings: 4

1 lb ground beef	½ cup breadcrumbs
½ cup onion, diced	Salt and black pepper to taste
1 egg	1 cup canned mushroom soup
½ tsp garlic powder	
½ cup Ricotta, crumbled	½ cup Colby cheese, grated
1 tbsp mixed dried herbs	

DIRECTIONS and Cooking Time: 30 Minutes
In a bowl, combine all ingredients, except for soup and colby cheese. Mix well with hands and shape into 4 meatballs. Coat the pressure cooker with spray. Add the meatballs and brown on all sides for a few minutes on Sauté. Pour in ½ cup of water and mushroom soup, seal the lid, and cook for 20 minutes on Manual at High. Do a quick pressure release. Stir in Colby cheese. Cook for 3 minutes on Sauté. Serve immediately.

Pork Chops With Veggies

INGREDIENTS for Servings: 6

6 bone-in, pork chops	1 tbsp canola oil
1 onion, chopped	2 tsp dried oregano, crushed
½ cup carrots, chopped	
¼ cup balsamic vinaigrette	1 (14 ½-oz) can diced tomatoes, drained

DIRECTIONS and Cooking Time: 45 Minutes
Set your IP to Sauté and heat canola oil. Add the pork chops and cook on both sides for about 5 minutes. Set aside. Add the carrots and onions and sauté for 4-6 minutes. Stir in the remaining ingredients and combine well. Return the chops and mix. Pour in 1 cup of water. Seal the lid, select Manual at High, and cook for 15 minutes. Release the pressure quickly. Serve warm.

Country Beef Stew With Sweet Potatoes

INGREDIENTS for Servings: 6

1 onion, diced	1 tsp garlic, minced
2 sweet potatoes, cubed	1 ½ cups vegetable broth
1 tbsp basil, chopped	3 tbsp tomato paste
1 tbsp parsley, chopped	1 bell pepper, chopped
1 tbsp oregano, chopped	1 tbsp canola oil
2 lb stewed beef meat, cubed	Salt and black pepper to taste

DIRECTIONS and Cooking Time: 45 Minutes
Heat oil on Sauté. Add bell pepper and onion and cook for about 3 minutes. Stir in garlic and cook for another minute. Add the beef and cook until browned on all sides. Stir in the remaining ingredients. Seal the lid and cook on Manual at High for 30 minutes. When it goes off, do a quick pressure release. Serve.

Chorizo With Bell Peppers & Onions

INGREDIENTS for Servings: 8

8 chorizo pork sausages	½ cup vegetable broth
2 onions, sliced	¼ cup white wine
4 red bell peppers, sliced	1 tsp garlic, minced
	Salt and black pepper to taste
1 tbsp olive oil	

DIRECTIONS and Cooking Time: 20 Minutes
On Sauté, heat oil, add sausages and brown for 5 minutes. Remove to a plate. Stir in onions and peppers. Stir-fry for 5 minutes until soft. Add garlic and cook for a minute. Add back the sausages and pour in broth and wine. Seal the lid and cook for 5 minutes on Manual at High. Once done, do a quick pressure release. Serve.

Pork Steaks With Apricot Sauce

INGREDIENTS for Servings: 4

4 pork steaks	¼ cup heavy cream
¼ cup milk	1 tbsp fruit jelly
8 apricots, pitted	½ tsp ground ginger
½ cup white wine	Salt and black pepper to taste
2 apples, peeled and sliced	

DIRECTIONS and Cooking Time: 25 Minutes
Place all ingredients, except for the jelly, in the pressure cooker. Stir to combine well and season with salt and pepper. Seal the lid and cook on Manual at High for 15 minutes. Once done, wait 5 minutes and do a quick pressure release. Stir in the jelly, serve, and enjoy.

Pear Pork Tenderloin

INGREDIENTS for Servings: 4

1 ¼ lb pork tenderloin	½ cup pear juice
1 chopped celery stalk	½ cup water
2 cups pears, chopped	¼ cup onions, chopped
1 cup cherries, pitted	
	Salt and black pepper to taste
	2 tbsp olive oil

DIRECTIONS and Cooking Time: 55 Minutes
Heat oil on Sauté and cook onions and celery for 5 minutes. Season the pork with salt and pepper, and add to the pot. Brown for 2-3 minutes per side. Top

with pears and cherries, and pour ½ cup water and pear juice. Seal the lid and cook on Manual for 40 minutes at High. Once ready, do a quick pressure release. Slice the pork tenderloin and arrange on a Servings platter. Spoon pear-cheery sauce over the pork and serve.

Pork Shoulder Infused With Lime & Mint

INGREDIENTS for Servings: 6

3 lb pork shoulder roast	½ cup fresh mint leaves
4 cloves garlic, minced	1 cup chopped cilantro
Salt and black pepper to taste	1 tbsp lime juice and zest
1 tbsp olive oil	Green onions, chopped

DIRECTIONS and Cooking Time: 75 Minutes
Mix together the ingredients in a bowl, except for the pork shoulder and mint leaves. Cover the pork shoulder with the paste and allow to marinate overnight. Arrange the mint leaves at the bottom of the IP and lay the marinated pork on top. Add 2 cups of water. Seal the lid, select Manual at High, and cook for 50 minutes. When ready, release the pressure naturally for 10 minutes. Remove and discard the mint leaves. Slice the meat and serve hot, topped with cooking sauce and freshly chopped green onions.

Fall Pork Loin Chops With Red Cabbage

INGREDIENTS for Servings: 4

4 pork loin chops, boneless	½ cup celery, chopped
4 cups red cabbage, pickled	2 onions, sliced
1 cup dry white wine	2 cups vegetable stock
2 cloves garlic, crushed	2 tsp mustard
1 cup carrots, chopped	Salt and black pepper to taste
	½ tsp chili powder
	½ cup tomato puree

DIRECTIONS and Cooking Time: 40 Minutes
Place the pork at the bottom of the pressure cooker. Add pickled cabbage on top. Add in the remaining ingredients and seal the lid. Select Manual and cook for 30 minutes at High. Once cooking is done, do a quick pressure release. Serve immediately.

Pork Chops In Cream Of Mushrooms

INGREDIENTS for Servings: 4

10 oz condensed cream of mushroom soup	1 cup milk
Salt and black pepper to taste	4 boneless pork chops
	1 tbsp ranch dressing

DIRECTIONS and Cooking Time: 35 Minutes
Combine all the ingredients, except for the pork chops, in a mixing bowl. Place the chops into the IP, and pour mixture over. Pour in ½ cup of water. Seal the lid, select Manual at High, and cook for 10 minutes. When ready, release the pressure naturally for 10 minutes.

Pork Sandwiches

INGREDIENTS for Servings: 6

2 lb boneless pork loin roast	1 ½ cups mango chutney
2 tbsp curry powder spice	6 hamburger buns
1 cup chicken broth	1 cup mayonnaise
	1 cup ketchup

DIRECTIONS and Cooking Time: 50 Minutes
Rub the outside of pork with curry powder. Add pork to the IP and pour in the chicken broth and mango chutney. Seal the lid, select Manual at High, and cook for 20 minutes. When ready, release the pressure quickly. Shred pork with two forks. Serve on buns with ketchup and mayonnaise.

Thyme Braised Lamb Shanks

INGREDIENTS for Servings: 4

4 lamb shanks	¼ cup plus 4 tsp flour
3 carrots, sliced	8 tsp olive oil
2 cups canned tomato, diced	1 onion, chopped
1 tbsp thyme	¾ cup red wine
1 garlic clove, crushed	¼ cup beef broth
1 tbsp chopped fresh oregano	Salt and black pepper to taste

DIRECTIONS and Cooking Time: 55 Minutes
In a plastic bag, place lamb shanks and ¼ cup of the flour. Shake until the shanks are well coated. Discard excess flour. In your IP, heat 4 tbsp oil on Sauté, and brown shanks on both sides. Remove to a plate. Add the remaining olive oil and sauté onion, garlic, and carrots for 4 minutes. Stir in tomatoes, wine, broth, thyme, and oregano. Return the shanks to the cooker. Seal the lid, select Manual at High, and set the timer to 40 minutes. When it beeps, do a quick pressure release. Whisk together the remaining flour and 8 tsp of cold water. Stir this mixture into the lamb sauce and cook until it thickens on Sauté. Serve immediately.

Beef & Tomato Curry

INGREDIENTS for Servings: 4

1 lb beef stew meat	1 onion, chopped
2 tbsp olive oil	1 jalapeño pepper, chopped
4 cups beef broth	1 tbsp curry powder
1 can (14.5-oz) tomatoes	Salt and black pepper to taste
1 tsp fresh ginger, minced	

DIRECTIONS and Cooking Time: 48 Minutes
Set your IP to Sauté and heat oil. Season the beef with salt and pepper. Cook for about 5 minutes on both sides until brown; set aside. Sauté curry powder, jalapeño pepper, onion, garlic, and ginger for 3 minutes. Stir in the tomatoes and broth. Seal the lid, select Manual at High, and cook for 20 minutes. When ready, do a quick release. Serve hot.

Winter Beef With Vegetables
INGREDIENTS for Servings: 4

5 oz pumpkin puree	1 cup mushrooms, sliced
3 tbsp olive oil	3 cups beef stock
2 carrots, chopped	Salt and black pepper to taste
½ tsp thyme	1 onion, sliced
1 garlic clove, minced	1 turnip, cubed
1 parsnip, chopped	½ tsp garlic powder
1 lb stewing beef meat, cubed	Chopped parsley for garnish
1 ½ cups green beans	

DIRECTIONS and Cooking Time: 40 Minutes
Heat olive oil on Sauté in the IP. Add the onion, carrots, parsnip, mushrooms, turnip, meat, and garlic, and cook for 5 minutes. Pour in the remaining ingredients and stir to combine. Seal the lid, select Manual at High, and cook for 20 minutes. Do a quick release. Serve the stew hot and sprinkle with freshly chopped parsley.

Ribs With Plum Sauce
INGREDIENTS for Servings: 4

1 tbsp soy sauce	2 tbsp cornstarch
¼ cup orange juice	½ cup honey
1 jar (7-oz) plum sauce	3 lb pork ribs, cut into Servings

DIRECTIONS and Cooking Time: 55 Minutes
Arrange the ribs inside the IP, add the plum sauce, soy sauce, honey, and a cup of water over the ribs. Seal the lid, select Manual at High, and cook for 25 minutes. When ready, release the pressure naturally for 10 minutes. Transfer the ribs to a plate and cover to keep warm. Set the IP to Sauté mode and add orange juice, and cornstarch and stir for a few minutes until well combined. Pour the sauce over the ribs and serve.

Juniper Beef Ragu
INGREDIENTS for Servings: 6

18 oz beef stew meat, cubed	3 juniper berries
2 bay leaves	1 tbsp parsley, chopped
5 garlic cloves, crushed	1 tsp cilantro
7 oz jarred roasted red peppers	½ cup beef broth
28 oz tomatoes, chopped	½ tbsp olive oil
	Salt and black pepper to taste

DIRECTIONS and Cooking Time: 65 Minutes
Season the beef with salt and pepper. Heat the oil on Sauté, and place the beef inside. Cook until the meat is browned on all sides. Chop red peppers and add along with the rest of the ingredients; stir to combine. Seal the lid, select Manual, and cook for 45 minutes at High. When ready, wait for the valve to drop on its own for a natural pressure release, for about 10 minutes. Serve.

Asian-style Flank Steaks
INGREDIENTS for Servings: 4

2 lb beef flank steak	1 cup water
2 tbsp olive oil	2/3 cup soy sauce
2 garlic cloves, minced	2 tbsp flour
1 cup carrots, grated	¾ cup Teriyaki sauce

DIRECTIONS and Cooking Time: 45 Minutes
Coat the beef in the flour and brown in heated olive oil on Sauté in the IP. Add in the remaining ingredients. Seal the lid, select Manual at High, and cook for 15 minutes. When ready, release the pressure naturally for 10 minutes. Serve hot.

Pork City Pot
INGREDIENTS for Servings: 6

1 lb stewing pork meat, cubed	1 (4-oz) can tomato sauce
4 potatoes, cubed	10.75 oz cream celery soup
Worcestershire sauce to taste	3 stalks celery, chopped
2 bay leaves	3 carrots, peeled and chopped
½ packet onion soup mix	

DIRECTIONS and Cooking Time: 45 Minutes
Place the meat and chopped vegetables into your IP. Dilute the cans of soup according to the instructions on the can. Combine them with dry soup mix and tomato sauce. Then pour over food in the cooker, and top with bay leaves. Pour in 1 cup of water. Seal the lid, select Manual at High, and cook for 20 minutes. When ready, release the pressure naturally for 5 minutes. Remove bay leaves. Serve the stew with fresh garlic bread.

Garlicky Bbq Pork Butt

INGREDIENTS for Servings: 6

2 lb pork butt	¼ tsp cumin powder
¼ tsp garlic powder	1 tsp rosemary
Salt and black pepper to taste	½ tsp onion powder
1 cup barbecue sauce	1 ½ cups vegetable broth

DIRECTIONS and Cooking Time: 55 Minutes
In a bowl, combine the barbecue sauce and all the spices. Brush the pork with the mixture. Press Sauté and coat the pot with cooking oil. Add pork and sear on all sides for 8 minutes. Pour the broth around the meat. Seal the lid and cook for 40 minutes on Manual at High. When ready, wait for 5 minutes before quick-releasing the pressure.

Sausage With Beer & Sauerkraut

INGREDIENTS for Servings: 6

2 lb kielbasa sausage, sliced	Salt and black pepper to taste
1 (12-oz) bottle beer	1 (20-oz) can sauerkraut
1 can (14-oz) tomatoes	2 tbsp parsley, chopped
1 tbsp paprika	
3 tbsp olive oil	

DIRECTIONS and Cooking Time: 41 Minutes
Heat olive oil on Sauté in the IP and cook the sausage for 5 minutes. Stir in paprika, salt, and pepper. Add in the remaining ingredients and stir. Pour in 1 cup of water, seal the lid, select Manual at High, and cook for 11 minutes. When ready, release the pressure naturally for 10 minutes. Serve hot topped with parsley.

Mexican-style Ropa Vieja

INGREDIENTS for Servings: 6

3 lb beef chuck roast	3 tomatoes, chopped
2 cups vegetable broth	1 tsp jalapeño powder
3 cloves garlic, minced	3 cups white rice, cooked
2 limes juiced	Salt and black pepper to taste
1 bay leaf	3 tbsp fresh cilantro, chopped
1 onion, sliced	

DIRECTIONS and Cooking Time: 64 Minutes
Set your IP to Sauté and heat olive oil. Add onion, garlic, tomatoes, and bay leaves and sauté for 3-4 minutes, stirring often. Pour in broth and beef. Season with salt, pepper, and jalapeño powder. Cover with water. Seal the lid, select Manual at High, and cook for 40 minutes. When ready, release the pressure naturally for 10 minutes. Remove the beef. Shred with two forks and return to the pot. Stir in the lime juice and discard bay leaf. Serve over white rice, sprinkled with cilantro.

POULTRY RECIPES

Chicken Fricassee
INGREDIENTS for Servings: 4

4 chicken breasts	½ cup dry white wine
2 tbsp olive oil	½ cup chicken broth
1 onion, chopped	¼ cup heavy cream
2 garlic cloves, minced	2 tbsp capers
Salt and black pepper to taste	1 bay leaf
	2 tbsp tarragon, chopped

DIRECTIONS and Cooking Time: 30 Minutes
Warm the olive oil in your Electric Pressure Cooker on Sauté. Sprinkle chicken with salt and pepper and place in the pot. Cook for 6 minutes on all sides. Add in onion and garlic and cook for 3 minutes. Pour in chicken broth, white wine, and bay leaf. Seal the lid, select Manual, and cook for 15 minutes on High pressure. When ready, perform a quick pressure release. Remove bay leaf and put in heavy cream and capers. Stir for 2-3 minutes and cook in the residual heat until thoroughly warmed. Ladle into bowls, top with tarragon, and serve.

Fettuccine With Duck Ragout
INGREDIENTS for Servings: 4

1 pound duck legs	1/2 cup tomato purée
2 sweet peppers, deseeded and finely chopped	1 red chili pepper, minced
2 cloves garlic, crushed	1/2 cup chicken bone broth
2 tablespoons dry cooking wine	1 pound fettuccine
1 onion, chopped	Sea salt and freshly ground black pepper, to taste

DIRECTIONS and Cooking Time: 30 Minutes
Bring a pot of salted water to a boil. Cook the fettuccine, stirring occasionally, until al dente. Drain, reserving 1 cup of the pasta water; set aside. Add the reserved pasta water along with the duck legs to the Electric Pressure Cooker. Secure the lid. Choose the "Manual" mode and cook for 20 minutes at High pressure. Once cooking is complete, use a quick pressure release; carefully remove the lid. Shred the meat with two forks. Add the meat back to the Electric Pressure Cooker. Add the remaining ingredients and press the "Sauté" button. Let it cook for 5 to 7 minutes more or until everything is heated through. Serve with the reserved pasta and enjoy!

Chicken Curry (ver. 1)
INGREDIENTS for Servings: 4

2 lbs chicken breast or thighs	6 oz can tomato paste
16 oz canned coconut milk	1 cup onion, chopped or ¼ cup dry minced onion
16 oz canned tomato sauce	2 tbsp curry powder
2 cloves garlic, minced	3 tbsp honey
	1 tsp salt

DIRECTIONS and Cooking Time: 40 Minutes
Combine all of the ingredients, except for the chicken, in the Electric Pressure Cooker and stir to combine. Add the chicken. Close and lock the lid. Select the MANUAL setting and set the cooking time for 15 minutes at HIGH pressure. Once cooking is complete, let the pressure Release Naturally for 15 minutes. Release any remaining steam manually. Open the lid and gently stir. Serve with cooked rice, potato or peas.

Allspice Turkey Drumsticks With Beer
INGREDIENTS for Servings: 2

1 lb. turkey drumsticks, boneless	¼ tsp. ground allspice
1 (6-oz) bottle beer	Sea salt and freshly ground black pepper, to taste
1 carrot, sliced	
1 small leek, sliced	

DIRECTIONS and Cooking Time: 20 Minutes
Place all the ingredients in the Electric Pressure Cooker and stir well. Lock the lid. Select the Manual mode and cook for 20 minutes at High Pressure. Once cooking is complete, do a natural pressure release for 10 minutes, then release any remaining pressure. Carefully open the lid. Remove from the pot and serve on a plate.

Simple Chicken Thighs
INGREDIENTS for Servings: 2-4

1 lb chicken thighs	2 tsp lime zest
2 tbsp oil	1 tsp chili powder
4 cups chicken broth	½ cup tomato puree
1 tsp salt	1 tbsp sugar

DIRECTIONS and Cooking Time: 50 Minutes
Season the meat evenly with salt and chili powder on both sides. Warm oil on Sauté, and add the thighs. Briefly brown on both sides and then set aside. Add the tomato puree, sugar, and lime zest. Cook for 10 minutes to obtain a thick sauce. Add the chicken thighs and pour in the broth. Seal the lid and cook on Poultry mode for 20 minutes on High pressure. When done, do a quick release and serve.

Sweet Saucy Chicken
INGREDIENTS for Servings: 2-4

4 chicken breasts, boneless and skinless	2 tbsp honey
Salt and black pepper to taste	2 tbsp minced garlic
	½ cup chicken broth
2 tbsp olive oil	1 tbsp cornstarch
2 tbsp soy sauce	1 tbsp water
2 tbsp tomato paste	½ cup chives, chopped

DIRECTIONS and Cooking Time: 45 Minutes
Season the chicken with pepper and salt. Warm oil on Sauté. Add in chicken and cook for 5 minutes until browned. In a small bowl, mix garlic, soy sauce, honey, and tomato paste. Pour the mixture over the chicken. Stir in ½ cup broth. Seal the lid and cook on High Pressure for 12 minutes. Release the Pressure quickly. Set the chicken to a bowl. Mix water and cornstarch to create a slurry. Briskly stir the mixture into the sauce left in the pan for 2 minutes until thickened. Serve the chicken with sauce and chives.

Bell Pepper & Carrot Chicken Stew

INGREDIENTS for Servings: 2-4

1 lb chicken breasts, boneless, skinless, cut into pieces	2 carrots, chopped
	1 tomato, roughly chopped
2 potatoes, peeled, chopped	A handful of freshly chopped parsley
5 green bell peppers, chopped, seeds removed	3 tbsp extra virgin olive oil
	1 tsp freshly ground chili pepper
2 ½ cups chicken broth	1 tsp salt

DIRECTIONS and Cooking Time: 35 Minutes
Warm the oil on Sauté, and stir-fry bell peppers and carrots, for 3 minutes. Add potatoes, tomatoes, and parsley. Sprinkle with cayenne, and salt, and stir well. Top with the chicken, Pour in broth and seal the lid. Cook on High Pressure for 13 minutes. When ready, do a quick Pressure release, and serve hot.

Cheesy Chicken Tenders

INGREDIENTS for Servings: 2

1 tbsp. softened butter	¼ tsp. smoked paprika
1 lb. chicken tenders	
½ cup vegetable broth	½ cup Cottage cheese, crumbled
Sea salt and freshly ground black pepper, to taste	1 heaping tbsp. fresh chives, roughly chopped

DIRECTIONS and Cooking Time: 12 Minutes
Press the Sauté button on your Electric Pressure Cooker and melt the butter. Brown the chicken tenders for 2 to 3 minutes. Add the broth, salt, black pepper, and paprika to the pot and whisk well. Lock the lid. Select the Manual mode and set the cooking time for 8 minutes at High Pressure. Once cooking is complete, do a natural pressure release for 5 minutes, then release any remaining pressure. Carefully open the lid. Add the crumbled cheese to the pot, cover, and allow to sit for 5 minutes until melted. Sprinkle the fresh chives on top for garnish before serving.

Bacon And Cheese Quiche

INGREDIENTS for Servings: 4

1 cup water	1 cup ground sausage, cooked
6 large eggs, beaten	
½ cup almond or coconut milk	4 slices cooked and crumbled bacon
¼ tsp salt	1 cup parmesan Cheese
1/8 tsp black pepper, ground	2 large green onions, chopped
½ cup diced ham	

DIRECTIONS and Cooking Time: 50 Minutes
Pour the water into the Electric Pressure Cooker and insert a steam rack. In a bowl, whisk together the eggs, milk, salt and pepper until combined. Add the ham, sausage, bacon, cheese and green onion and stir well. Cover the dish with foil and place on the steam rack. Close and lock the lid. Select MANUAL and cook at HIGH pressure for 30 minutes. Once cooking is complete, use a Natural Release for 10 minutes, then release any remaining pressure manually. Uncover the pot. Remove the foil. Serve. If you like a crisp top, you can sprinkle the dish with some additional cheese then slide under the broiler for a few minutes at the end.

Chicken With Black Beans

INGREDIENTS for Servings: 4

1 small onion chopped	½ cup water
4 cups diced tomatoes with juice	2 teaspoons sea salt.
	½ teaspoon ground black pepper
2 lbs boneless, skinless chicken breasts	2 tablespoons butter.
	1 can organic black beans drained and rinsed
1 tablespoon chipotle peppers	
1 cup jasmine rice uncooked ½ lime, juiced	2 cups cheddar chesses for serving, shredded

DIRECTIONS and Cooking Time: 6 Minutes
Put the chicken, tomatoes, peppers, water, rice, salt, lemon juice, butter and onion in your Electric Pressure Cooker. Use 'manual' settings on high pressure for 6 minutes. Let it cook until the cooker beeps. Use the 'quick pressure release' to vent the steam. Add the black beans to the chicken then stir well. Add the salt and pepper to taste. Serve with shredded cheese on top.

Salsa Verde Chicken

INGREDIENTS for Servings: 6

2½ lbs boneless chicken breasts 1 tsp smoked paprika 1 tsp cumin	1 tsp salt 2 cup (16 oz) salsa verde

DIRECTIONS and Cooking Time: 25 Minutes
Add the chicken breasts, paprika, cumin, and salt to the Electric Pressure Cooker. Pour the salsa verde on top. Close and lock the lid. Select the MANUAL setting and set the cooking time for 20 minutes at HIGH pressure. Once pressure cooking is complete, use a Quick Release. Unlock and carefully open the lid. Shred the meat. Serve.

Pilaf With Zucchini & Chicken

INGREDIENTS for Servings: 4

2 tsp olive oil 1 zucchini, chopped 2 garlic cloves, minced 1 tbsp chopped fresh rosemary 2 tsp chopped fresh thyme leaves	1 cup leeks, chopped Salt and black pepper to taste 2 cups chicken stock 1 lb boneless, skinless chicken legs 1 cup rice, rinsed

DIRECTIONS and Cooking Time: 40 Minutes
Warm oil on Sauté, add in zucchini and cook for 5 minutes until tender. Stir in thyme, leeks, rosemary, pepper, salt and garlic. Cook the mixture for 3-4 minutes. Add ½ cup chicken stock into the pot to deglaze, scrape the bottom to get rid of any browned bits of food. When liquid stops simmering, add in the remaining stock, rice, and chicken with more pepper and salt. Seal the lid and cook on High Pressure for 5 minutes. Do a quick release.

Orange & Red Pepper Infused Chicken

INGREDIENTS for Servings: 4

2 tsp red pepper flakes 1 cup orange-tangerine juice 1/3 cup honey	4 chicken breasts, halved Salt and black pepper to taste Chopped cilantro for garnish

DIRECTIONS and Cooking Time: 35 Minutes
Coat your IP with cooking spray and add in the chicken breasts. In a bowl, mix together the remaining ingredients until well combined. Pour the mixture over the chicken breasts along with a cup of water. Seal the lid, select Manual at High, and cook for 20 minutes. When ready, release the pressure naturally for 5 minutes. Serve hot, sprinkled with flesh cilantro.

Drumsticks In Adobo Sauce

INGREDIENTS for Servings: 2-4

1 lb chicken drumsticks ½ cup plain vinegar ½ cup soy sauce 1 bay leaf 2 tbsp olive oil 10 Ancho dried chilies, seeds removed 5 Guajillo dried chilies, seeds removed	8 garlic cloves, peeled ½ tsp Mexican oregano ½ tsp cumin powder A pinch clove powder Salt and black pepper to taste ¼ cup apple cider vinegar ½ cup water 2 tbsp chopped cilantro to garnish

DIRECTIONS and Cooking Time: 35 Min + Marinating Time
In a medium bowl, combine chicken, vinegar, soy sauce, and bay leaf. Cover the bowl with a plastic wrap and marinate chicken in the fridge for 1 hour. Set your Electric Pressure Cooker to Sauté. Remove chicken from marinade, and fry in olive oil on both sides until golden brown, 6 minutes. Transfer to a paper towel-lined plate and set aside. Meanwhile, in a blender, grind chilies, garlic, oregano, cumin powder, and clove powder until smooth paste forms. Pour mixture into the oil in inner pot and stir-fry until fragrant, 3 minutes. Add salt, black pepper, vinegar, and water; stir and arrange chicken in the sauce. Seal the lid, select Manual on High, and set cooking time to 4 minutes. After cooking, perform natural pressure release for 10 minutes. Spoon chicken with sauce into serving bowls and garnish with cilantro. Serve warm with rice.

Turkey Stew With Root Vegetables

INGREDIENTS for Servings: 4

1 pound turkey legs 1/2 teaspoon Hungarian paprika 2 tablespoons fresh cilantro leaves, chopped 1 red bell pepper, chopped 1 parsnip, chopped 1/2 pound carrots, chopped 1/2 cup leeks, chopped	1 cup turnip, chopped 2 garlic cloves, minced 1 green bell pepper, chopped 1 Serrano pepper, chopped Sea salt and ground black pepper, to taste 2 tablespoons butter, at room temperature 2 cups turkey stock

DIRECTIONS and Cooking Time: 20 Minutes
Press the "Sauté" button to preheat your Electric Pressure Cooker and melt the butter. Now, sear the turkey, skin side down, 3 minutes on each side. Sprinkle the turkey legs with salt and black pepper as you cook them. Stir the remaining ingredients into the Electric Pressure Cooker. Secure the lid and select the "Manual" mode. Cook for 15 minutes at High pressure. Once cooking is complete, use a natural pressure release. Transfer the turkey legs to a bowl

and let them cool. Then, strip the meat off the bones, cut it into small pieces and return to the Electric Pressure Cooker. Serve hot and enjoy!

Creamy Chicken With Tomato Sauce

INGREDIENTS for Servings: 2

2 chicken drumsticks	1 tsp garlic paste
2 cups tomato sauce	Salt and black pepper to taste
1 cup heavy cream	½ tsp rosemary, chopped
1 cup Pecorino Romano, grated	½ tsp fresh thyme, chopped
4 tbsp butter	
1 tbsp basil leaves, chopped	

DIRECTIONS and Cooking Time: 35 Minutes
Melt butter on Sauté in IP. Add garlic paste, tomato sauce, rosemary, thyme, and basil. Sprinkle chicken drumsticks with salt and pepper. Place drumsticks on top of the sauce, so it resembles a nestle. Seal the lid, select Poultry, and cook at High for 20 minutes. Once done, release pressure naturally for 5 minutes. Stir in cheese and heavy cream and serve right away.

Homemade Turkey Burgers

INGREDIENTS for Servings: 2-4

1 lb ground turkey	1 cup flour
2 eggs	½ tsp salt
1 onion, finely chopped	½ tsp black pepper, ground
2 tsp dried dill, chopped	1 cup sour cream

DIRECTIONS and Cooking Time: 25 Minutes
In a bowl, add all ingredients and mix well with hands. Form the patties with the previously prepared mixture. Line parchment paper over a baking dish and arrange the patties. Pour 1 cup of water in the pot. Lay the trivet and place the baking dish on top. Seal the lid. Cook on Pressure Cook mode for 15 minutes on High. Release the pressure naturally, for 10 minutes. Serve with lettuce and tomatoes.

Rich Meatball Soup

INGREDIENTS for Servings: 6

2 teaspoons sesame oil	1 cup tomato puree
1 pound cavatappi pasta	Sea salt and ground black pepper, to your liking
2 tablespoons fresh coriander, chopped	1 pound ground turkey
1 celery with leaves, chopped	1/2 pound ground pork
1/2 white onion, finely chopped	1 teaspoon dill weed
2 garlic cloves, minced	1 carrot, thinly sliced
	6 cups chicken stock
1 tablespoon oyster sauce	1 teaspoon cayenne pepper
	1 whole egg

DIRECTIONS and Cooking Time: 20 Minutes
Thoroughly combine the ground meat, coriander, onion, garlic, oyster sauce, salt, black pepper, and cayenne pepper. Shape the mixture into meatballs; set aside. Press the "Sauté" button to heat up the Electric Pressure Cooker. Heat the oil and sear the meatballs until they are browned on all sides. Now, stir in the remaining ingredients. Secure the lid. Choose the "Manual" setting and cook for 12 minutes under High pressure. Once cooking is complete, use a quick pressure release; carefully remove the lid. Bon appétit!

Lemony Chicken With Red Currants

INGREDIENTS for Servings: 6

1 ½ lb chicken breasts	1 cup kalamata olives, pitted
¼ cup red currants	2 tbsp sesame oil
2 garlic cloves, minced	1 tsp coriander seeds
6 lemon slices	1 tsp cumin
1 cup green onions	Salt and black pepper to taste

DIRECTIONS and Cooking Time: 35 Minutes
Heat oil on Sauté. Add green onions, coriander seeds, and garlic and cook for 3 minutes. Add chicken and top with olives and red currants. Season with salt and pepper. Arrange the lemon slices on top, and pour 2 ¼ cups of water over. Seal the lid and cook on Poultry for 15 minutes at High. When ready, release pressure naturally for 10 minutes. Serve.

Spring Onion Buffalo Wings

INGREDIENTS for Servings: 6

2 lb chicken wings, sectioned	3 tbsp butter
½ cup hot pepper sauce	Sea salt to taste
	2 tbsp sugar, light brown
1 tbsp Worcestershire sauce	2 spring onions, sliced diagonally

DIRECTIONS and Cooking Time: 25 Minutes
Combine hot sauce, Worcestershire sauce, butter, salt, and brown sugar in a bowl and microwave for 20 seconds until the butter melts. Pour 1 cup of water in your Electric Pressure Cooker and fit in a trivet. Place the chicken wings on the trivet and seal the lid. Select Manual and cook for 10 minutes on High pressure. Once done, perform a quick pressure release and unlock the lid. Remove chicken wings to a baking dish and brush the top with marinade. Broil for 4-5 minutes, turn the wings and brush more marinade.

Broil for 4-5 minutes more. Top with spring onions and serve.

Tender Chicken With Garden Vegetables

INGREDIENTS for Servings: 4

2 tablespoons lard, at room temperature	1/2 cup leeks, sliced
1 pound chicken breasts, sliced into serving-size pieces	2 garlic cloves, sliced
	1 cup chicken bone broth
1 teaspoon dried marjoram	2 cups butternut squash, diced
1/2 teaspoon dried sage	1 eggplant, diced
	1/2 head cabbage, diced
1/2 teaspoon ground black pepper	1/4 cup fresh chives, chopped
Sea salt, to taste	

DIRECTIONS and Cooking Time: 20 Minutes
Press the "Sauté" button and melt the lard until sizzling. Then, sear the chicken breasts until it is lightly browned or about 5 minutes. Add the spices and stir to combine. Add the leeks and garlic. Pour in the chicken bone broth. Afterwards, add the vegetables and secure the lid. Choose the "Manual" mode. Cook for 8 minutes at High pressure. Once cooking is complete, use a quick pressure release; carefully remove the lid. Using a slotted spoon, remove the chicken and vegetables to a serving platter. Press the "Sauté" button and simmer the cooking liquid for about 3 minutes until slightly thickened. Serve garnished with fresh chives. Bon appétit!

Savory Chicken Wings With Worcestershire Sauce

INGREDIENTS for Servings: 8

8 chicken wings, bones and skin on	1/3 cup Worcestershire sauce
3 cups chicken broth	2 spring onions, finely chopped
1 tsp fresh ginger, grated	2 garlic cloves, crushed
1 tbsp honey	
2 tbsp oil	1 tsp salt

DIRECTIONS and Cooking Time: 35 Minutes
Add the chicken to the pot and pour in broth. Seal the lid and cook on Poultry for 15 minutes on High. Do a quick release. Remove chicken and broth, and wipe the pot clean. Heat oil on Sauté, and stir-fry onions and garlic for 2-3 minutes. Add Worcestershire sauce, honey, salt, and ginger. Cook for a minute and return the wings. Stir well and cook for 2 minutes, until nice and crispy.

Creamed Taco Chicken Salad

INGREDIENTS for Servings: 5

1 bell pepper, sliced	1 cup green onions, sliced
1/2 cup radishes, sliced	
1 cucumber, chopped	1 carrot, shredded
1/2 teaspoon taco seasoning	2 chicken breasts, boneless and skinless
1 teaspoon Dijon mustard	2 tablespoons cilantro, chopped
1 cup frozen corn, thawed	1 sprig rosemary
	1/2 cup sour cream
1 sprig thyme	1/2 cup mayonnaise
1 sprig sage	Seasoned salt and ground black pepper, to taste
2 garlic cloves, pressed	

DIRECTIONS and Cooking Time: 15 Minutes
Add 1 ½ cups of water and a metal trivet to your Electric Pressure Cooker. Then, season the chicken breast with salt, black pepper and taco seasoning. Place the seasoned chicken breast onto the trivet. Top with thyme, rosemary, sage, and garlic. Now, secure the lid. Choose the "Poultry" setting and cook for 5 minutes under High pressure. Once cooking is complete, use a natural pressure release; carefully remove the lid. Allow the chicken to cool and cut it into strips. Stir in the remaining ingredients; gently stir to combine well. Serve well-chilled.

Mom's Orange Chicken

INGREDIENTS for Servings: 4

1 tablespoon olive oil	1 medium red onion, chopped
2/3 pound ground chicken	2 garlic cloves, minced
1/3 pound bacon, chopped	1 jalapeno pepper, chopped
2 tablespoons sherry wine	1 teaspoon paprika
	Fresh juice and zest of 1/2 orange
Sea salt and ground black pepper, to taste	1 tablespoon arrowroot powder

DIRECTIONS and Cooking Time: 15 Minutes
Press the "Sauté" button and heat the oil until sizzling. Sear the chicken and bacon until they are slightly brown. Add the sherry wine and stir with a wooden spoon, scraping up the browned bits on the bottom of the pan. Add the red onion, garlic, and jalapeno pepper; stir to combine. Season with salt, black pepper, and paprika. Pour in 1 cup of water. Secure the lid. Choose "Poultry" mode. Cook for 5 minutes at High pressure. Once cooking is complete, use a quick pressure release; carefully remove the lid. Add the orange juice and zest; stir in the arrowroot powder. Press the "Sauté" button and simmer, stirring occasionally, until it thickens. Bon appétit!

Chicken With Port Wine Sauce

INGREDIENTS for Servings: 6

1 (3 lb) chicken, cut into pieces	¼ cup Port wine
2 tbsp olive oil	Salt and black pepper to taste
1 large onion, finely diced	2 tbsp parsley, chopped
1 cup mushrooms	

DIRECTIONS and Cooking Time: 35 Minutes
Warm olive oil in your IP on Sauté. Add in the chicken pieces and cook until the chicken is light brown, about 6-7 minutes; set aside. Add onion and mushrooms to the pot and sauté for 3-4 minutes. Deglaze with Port wine and pour in 1 cup of water. Season with salt and pepper and return the chicken. Seal the lid, select Manual, and cook for 20 minutes on High. Once ready, release pressure naturally for 10 minutes. Sprinkle with parsley and serve.

Chicken Drumsticks With Potatoes & Veggies

INGREDIENTS for Servings: 4

4 potatoes, peeled and quartered	2 tsp fresh oregano
4 cups water	3 tbsp finely chopped parsley
2 lemons, zested and juiced	1 cup packed watercress
1 tbsp olive oil	1 cucumber, sliced
1 tsp red pepper flakes	½ cup cherry tomatoes, quartered
Salt and black pepper to taste	¼ cup kalamata olives, pitted
2 serrano peppers, stemmed, cored, chopped	¼ cup hummus
	¼ cup feta cheese, crumbled
4 boneless skinless chicken drumsticks	Lemon wedges, for serving

DIRECTIONS and Cooking Time: 40 Minutes
In the cooker, add water and potatoes. Set trivet over them. In a baking bowl, mix lemon juice, olive oil, black pepper, oregano, zest, salt, and red pepper flakes. Add chicken drumsticks in the marinade and stir to coat. Set the bowl with chicken on the trivet in the inner pot. Seal the lid, select Poultry and cook on High for 15 minutes. Do a quick release. Take out the bowl with chicken and the trivet from the pot. Drain potatoes and add parsley and salt. Divide the potatoes between four serving plates and top with watercress, cucumber slices, hummus, cherry tomatoes, chicken, olives, and feta cheese. Garnish with lemon wedges to serve.

Cannellini & Sausage Stew

INGREDIENTS for Servings: 2

½ tbsp olive oil	⅓ sprig fresh sage
⅓ lb Italian sausages, halved	½ bay leaf
⅓ celery stalk, chopped	½ cup Cannellini beans, soaked and rinsed
⅓ carrot, chopped	3/4 cup vegetable stock
⅓ onion, chopped	1 cup fresh spinach
⅓ sprig fresh rosemary	⅓ tsp salt

DIRECTIONS and Cooking Time: 45 Minutes
Warm oil on Sauté. Add in sausage pieces and sear for 5 minutes until browned; set aside on a plate. To the pot, add celery, onion, bay leaf, sage, carrot, and rosemary; cook for 3 minutes to soften slightly. Stir in vegetable stock and beans. Arrange seared sausage pieces on top of the beans. Seal the lid, press Bean/Chili and cook on High for 10 minutes. Release Pressure naturally for 20 minutes, do a quick release. Get rid of bay leaf, rosemary and sage. Mix spinach into the mixture to serve.

Cumin Shredded Chicken

INGREDIENTS for Servings: 5

2 lb chicken thighs, boneless and skinless	1 tsp cumin, dried
2 tbsp olive oil	1 yellow onion, chopped
1 cup salsa verde	2 tbsp lime juice
1 tsp thyme, dried	Cilantro, chopped for garnish
Salt and black pepper to taste	3 cups white rice, cooked
2 garlic cloves, minced	

DIRECTIONS and Cooking Time: 43 Minutes
Heat oil on Sauté in the IP. Cook the chicken thighs for 5 minutes. Add salsa verde, thyme, garlic, onion, salt and pepper, and cook for 3 minutes. Pour in 2 cups of water. Seal the lid, select Manual at High, and cook for 20 minutes. When ready, do a quick release and remove the thighs to a plate. Shred the meat then return it to the IP. Serve over cooked rice, garnished with cilantro and lime juice.

Hard-boiled Eggs

INGREDIENTS for Servings: 4-8

5-15 eggs	1 cup water

DIRECTIONS and Cooking Time: 15 Minutes
Pour the water into the Electric Pressure Cooker and insert a steamer basket. Put the eggs in the basket. Close and lock the lid. Select MANUAL and cook at HIGH pressure for 5 minutes. Once timer goes off, allow to Naturally Release for 5 minutes. Then use a Quick Release. Transfer the eggs to the bowl of cold water. Wait 2-3 minutes. If you like, you can peel immediately

Chicken Congee

INGREDIENTS for Servings: 4-6

6 chicken drumsticks	½ cup scallions, chopped
7 cups water	
1 cup Jasmine rice	2 tbs sesame oil, optional
1 tbsp fresh ginger	
Salt to taste	

DIRECTIONS and Cooking Time: 65 Minutes
Rinse the rice well. Add the chicken, rice, water and ginger to the Electric Pressure Cooker. Stir well. Close and lock the lid. Select the MANUAL setting and set the cooking time for 25 minutes at HIGH pressure. Once cooking is complete, select CANCEL and let Naturally Release for 10 minutes. Release any remaining steam manually. Open the lid. Take the chicken out from the pot, shred the meat and discard the bones. Return the chicken meat to the pot. Select SAUTÉ and cook, stirring occasionally, for about 10 minutes, or until thickened. Top with scallions and sesame oil. Serve.

Chicken & Mushrooms With White Wine

INGREDIENTS for Servings: 4

1 (10.75-oz) can condensed mushroom soup	1 tbsp milk
	¼ tsp garlic powder
	¼ cup white wine
4 chicken breasts, halved	1 tsp parsley, dried
	1 tsp onion, dried, minced
Salt and black pepper to taste	
	Chopped chives for garnish
1 cup mushrooms, sliced	

DIRECTIONS and Cooking Time: 35 Minutes
Mix all the ingredients into your IP and stir to combine well. Pour in 1 cup of water. Seal the lid, select Manual at High, and cook for 20 minutes. When ready, release the pressure naturally for 5 minutes. Serve topped with freshly chopped chives.

Tarragon Whole Chicken

INGREDIENTS for Servings: 6

1 (3 lb) whole chicken	1 tbsp paprika
1 tsp tarragon, chopped	Salt and black pepper to taste
3 tbsp butter, softened	1 cup chicken broth
1 tbsp onion powder	1 tbsp white wine
1 tbsp garlic powder	2 tsp soy sauce
	1 minced green onion

DIRECTIONS and Cooking Time: 40 Minutes
Combine butter, tarragon, salt, onion powder, garlic powder, paprika, salt, and pepper in a bowl. Pour 1 cup of water, white wine, and soy sauce in your Electric Pressure Cooker and fit in a trivet. Brush chicken with butter mixture on all sides and place it on the trivet. Seal the lid, select Manual, and cook for 25 minutes on High pressure. When done, allow a natural release for 10 minutes and unlock the lid. Serve topped with minced green onion.

Easy Teriyaki Chicken

INGREDIENTS for Servings: 4

2 tablespoons sesame oil	1/4 cup brown sugar
	1 teaspoon ground ginger
1 pound chicken drumettes, skinless, boneless, cut into bite-sized chunks	2 tablespoons rice wine
	3 tablespoons Mirin
	1 pound broccoli florets
2 garlic cloves, minced	
1/4 cup soy sauce	
1/2 cup water	1 teaspoon arrowroot powder
1/2 cup rice vinegar	

DIRECTIONS and Cooking Time: 30 Minutes
Press the "Sauté" button to preheat your Electric Pressure Cooker. Heat the sesame oil and cook the chicken drumettes for 3 to 4 minutes. Then, add the garlic and cook for 30 seconds more or until fragrant. Add the soy sauce, water, vinegar, sugar, ginger, rice wine, and Mirin. Secure the lid. Choose the "Manual" mode and cook for 10 minutes at High pressure. Once cooking is complete, use a quick pressure release; carefully remove the lid. Add the broccoli florets and secure the lid. Choose the "Manual" mode and cook for 2 minutes at High pressure. Once cooking is complete, use a quick pressure release; carefully remove the lid. Transfer the chicken and broccoli to a nice serving platter. Press the "Sauté" button to preheat your Electric Pressure Cooker again. Add the arrowroot powder and stir until it is completely dissolved. Cook for 5 to 6 minutes or until the sauce thickens slightly. Spoon over the chicken and serve.

Pumpkin & Wild Rice Cajun Chicken

INGREDIENTS for Servings: 6

6 chicken thighs, skinless	2 tbsp olive oil
	1 cup pumpkin, peeled and cubed
Salt and white pepper to taste	
	2 celery stalks, diced
½ tsp ground red pepper	2 onions, diced
	2 garlic cloves, crushed
½ tsp onion powder	
1 tsp cajun seasoning	3 cups chicken broth
1/8 tsp smoked paprika	1 ½ cups wild rice

DIRECTIONS and Cooking Time: 45 Minutes
Season the chicken with salt, onion powder, cajun seasoning, white pepper, red pepper, and paprika. Warm oil on Sauté. Stir in celery and pumpkin and cook for 5 minutes until tender; set the vegetables on

a plate. In batches, sear chicken in oil for 3 minutes each side until golden brown; set on a plate. Into the cooker, add ¼ cup chicken stock to deglaze the pan, scrape away any browned bits from the bottom; add garlic and onion and cook for 2 minutes until fragrant. Take back the celery and pumpkin the cooker; add the wild rice and remaining chicken stock. Place the chicken over the rice mixture. Seal the lid and cook for 10 minutes on High Pressure. Release the Pressure quickly. Place rice and chicken pieces in serving plates and serve.

Juicy Turkey With Mushrooms
INGREDIENTS for Servings: 4

1 ½ lb turkey breast	1 garlic clove, minced
6 oz white button mushrooms, sliced	2 tbsp olive oil
3 tbsp leeks, chopped	3 tbsp whipping cream
½ tsp dried sage	1 ½ tbsp cornstarch
¼ cup dry white wine	Salt and black pepper to taste
⅔ cup chicken stock	

DIRECTIONS and Cooking Time: 35 Minutes
Warm half of olive oil on Sauté. Season with salt and pepper. Add turkey to the IP and cook for about 3 minutes on each side. Transfer to a plate. Heat the remaining oil and cook leeks, thyme, garlic, sage, and mushrooms. Add white wine to scrape off any brown bits at the bottom. When the alcohol evaporates, return the turkey to the cooker. Seal the lid and cook on Manual for 15 minutes at High. Do a quick pressure release. Combine whipping cream and cornstarch in a small bowl. Open the lid and stir in the mixture. Cook on Sauté, until the sauce thickens. Slice the turkey in half and serve topped with the creamy sauce.

Momma's Chicken With Salsa Verde
INGREDIENTS for Servings: 2-4

Salsa Verde:	¼ cup extra virgin olive oil
1 jalapeño pepper, deveined and chopped	Chicken:
½ cup capers	4 boneless skinless chicken breasts
¼ cup parsley	2 cups water
1 lime, juiced	1 cup quinoa, rinsed
1 tsp salt	

DIRECTIONS and Cooking Time: 50 Minutes
In a blender, mix olive oil, salt, lime juice, jalapeño pepper, capers, and parsley and blend until smooth. Arrange chicken breasts on the bottom of the cooker. Over the chicken, add salsa verde mixture. In a bowl that can fit in the cooker, mix quinoa and water. Set a steamer rack onto chicken and sauce. Set the bowl onto the rack. Seal the lid and cook on High Pressure for 20 minutes. Release the Pressure quickly. Remove the quinoa bowl and rack. Using two forks, shred chicken into the sauce; stir to coat. Divide the quinoa, between plates. Top with chicken and salsa verde before serving.

Country Chicken With Vegetables
INGREDIENTS for Servings: 4

4 boneless, skinless chicken thighs	1 chopped onion
Salt and black pepper to taste	1 tbsp tomato paste
	10-12 cherry tomatoes, halved
2 tbsp olive oil	½ cup pitted green olives
2 chopped carrots	
½ lb green peas	½ cup fresh basil, minced
1 cup quartered cremini mushrooms	
3 garlic cloves, smashed	¼ cup parsley, chopped

DIRECTIONS and Cooking Time: 25 Minutes
Sprinkle chicken thighs with salt and pepper. Warm the olive oil in your Electric Pressure Cooker on Sauté and cook carrots, mushrooms, and onion for 5 minutes. Add in garlic and tomato paste and cook for another 30 seconds. Stir in cherry tomatoes, chicken thighs, and olives. Pour in 1 cup of water. Seal the lid, select Manual, and cook for 10 minutes on High pressure. Once ready, perform a quick pressure release and unlock the lid. Select Sauté and mix in green peas; cook for 5 minutes. Serve topped with fresh basil and parsley.

Spicy Honey Chicken
INGREDIENTS for Servings: 4

4 chicken drumsticks	2 tbsp hot chili sauce
5 tbsp soy sauce	2 tbsp cornstarch
2 tbsp honey	1 lime, cut into wedges
1 cup chicken broth	
1 garlic clove, minced	

DIRECTIONS and Cooking Time: 20 Minutes
Place soy sauce, honey, garlic, and chili sauce in your Electric Pressure Cooker and stir. Add in chicken drumsticks and toss to coat. Pour in chicken broth and seal the lid. Select Manual and cook for 12 minutes on High pressure. Mix 2 tbsp of water and cornstarch in a bowl. When over, perform a quick pressure release and unlock the lid. Add in the slurry and simmer on Sauté until the sauce thickens. Serve right away.

Traditional Locrio De Pollo
INGREDIENTS for Servings: 5

5 ounces chorizo sausage, casings removed and crumbled	1 pound chicken breasts, trimmed and cut into bite-sized pieces
1 cup short-grain white rice	1/2 teaspoon saffron threads
1/2 cup brown onion,	5 ounces seafood mix

chopped 2 tablespoons fresh parsley, roughly chopped 1 ½ cups chicken broth 1 cup tomato puree 1 teaspoon dried oregano	2 tablespoons Rueda 1 lemon, juiced and zested 1 tablespoon olive oil Sea salt and ground black pepper, to taste

DIRECTIONS and Cooking Time: 20 Minutes
Press the "Sauté" button and heat the olive oil. Now, cook the brown onion and chicken until the onion is translucent and the chicken is no longer pink or about 4 minutes. Deglaze the pot with the Rueda wine. Stir in the rice, broth, tomato puree, oregano, salt, black pepper, and saffron. Secure the lid and choose the "Manual" mode. Cook for 5 minutes at High pressure. Afterwards, use a quick release and carefully remove the lid. Add the seafood mix and sausage. Secure the lid and choose the "Manual" mode. Cook for 4 to 5 minutes at High pressure; use a quick release and carefully remove the lid. Add the lemon and parsley and serve immediately. Bon appétit!

Cranberry Turkey With Hazelnuts

INGREDIENTS for Servings: 5

1 lb turkey breast, boneless, skinless, cut into thick slices 3 tbsp butter, softened 2 cups fresh cranberries 1 cup red wine	1 cup toasted hazelnuts, chopped 1 tbsp fresh rosemary, chopped 2 tbsp olive oil 2 tbsp orange zest Salt and black pepper to taste

DIRECTIONS and Cooking Time: 40 Minutes
Rub the turkey with oil and sprinkle with orange zest, salt, pepper, and rosemary. Melt butter in pot, and brown turkey breast for 5-6 minutes, on Sauté mode. Pour in wine, cranberries and 1 cup of water. Seal the lid. Cook on High Pressure for 25 minutes. Do a quick release. Serve with chopped hazelnuts.

Fabulous Orange Chicken Stew

INGREDIENTS for Servings: 4

2 lb chicken breast, boneless and skinless 1 cup fire-roasted tomatoes, diced 1 tbsp chili powder	Salt and white pepper to taste 1 cup orange juice 2 cups chicken broth

DIRECTIONS and Cooking Time: 50 Minutes
Season the chicken with salt and pepper, and place in your Electric Pressure Cooker. Add the remaining ingredients, except for the orange juice and chicken broth, and cook on Sauté mode for 10 minutes, stirring occasionally. Press Cancel, pour in the broth and orange juice. Seal the lid and cook on Poultry for 25 minutes on High. Release the pressure naturally, for 10 minutes. Serve immediately.

Asian Garlic And Honey Chicken

INGREDIENTS for Servings: 6

1 ½ pounds chicken breasts, cut into cubes 6 tablespoons honey 3 cloves of garlic, minced 2 tablespoons online powder 1 ½ tablespoons soy sauce	½ tablespoon sriracha sauce 1 cup water 1 tablespoon cornstarch + 2 tablespoons water Green onions, chopped 1 tablespoon sesame oil

DIRECTIONS and Cooking Time: 15 Minutes
Place all ingredients except for the cornstarch slurry and green onions in the Electric Pressure Cooker. Give a good stir. Close the lid and press the Poultry button.4. Adjust the cooking time to 15 minutes. Do quick pressure release. Once the lid is open, press the Sauté button and stir in the cornstarch slurry.7. Simmer until the sauce thickens. Stir in green onions and sesame oil last.

Chicken With Artichokes And Bacon

INGREDIENTS for Servings: 4

2 chicken breasts, skinless, boneless, and halved 2 cups canned artichokes, drained, and chopped 1 cup water	1 cup bacon, cooked and crumbled 2 tbsps. tomato paste 1 tbsp. chives, chopped Salt, to taste

DIRECTIONS and Cooking Time: 25 Minutes
Mix all the ingredients in your Electric Pressure Cooker until well combined. Lock the lid. Select the Poultry mode and set the cooking time for 25 minutes at High Pressure. Once cooking is complete, do a natural pressure release for 10 minutes, then release any remaining pressure. Carefully open the lid. Remove from the pot to a large plate and serve.

Buttered Chicken With Artichokes & Rosemary

INGREDIENTS for Servings: 3

1 lb chicken breasts, boneless, skinless, chopped 2 artichokes, trimmed, halved	1 lemon, juiced Salt and black pepper to taste 1 tbsp rosemary, chopped 1 cup water

2 tbsp butter, melted	
2 tbsp olive oil	

DIRECTIONS and Cooking Time: 35 Minutes
Heat oil on Sauté and cook the chicken for a minute per side, until slightly golden. Pour in 1 cup of water, seal the lid, and cook on High pressure for 13 minutes. Do a quick release. Set aside. Place the trivet and pour water. Rub the artichoke halves with half of the lemon juice, and arrange on top of the trivet. Seal the lid and cook on Steam for 3 minutes on High. Do a quick release. Combine artichoke and chicken in a large bowl. Stir in salt, pepper, and lemon juice. Drizzle butter over and sprinkle with rosemary to serve.

Easy Millet And Chicken Bowl

INGREDIENTS for Servings: 4

4 chicken drumsticks, skinless and boneless	1/2 teaspoon red pepper flakes, crushed
Sea salt and ground black pepper, to taste	1/2 cup shallots, chopped
1/2 teaspoon dried basil	2 garlic cloves, finely chopped
1/2 teaspoon dried oregano	1 bell pepper, deseeded and chopped
1/2 teaspoon ground cumin	1 cup millet
1 ½ tablespoons olive oil	1 cup vegetable broth
	1 cup tomato puree
	1 bay leaf
	1 cup green beans

DIRECTIONS and Cooking Time: 25 Minutes
Season the chicken drumsticks with salt, black pepper, red pepper, basil, oregano, and cumin. Press the "Sauté" button and heat the olive oil. Sear the chicken drumsticks for 5 minutes, turning them to ensure even cooking. Add the shallots, garlic, pepper, millet, broth, tomato puree, and bay leaf to the Electric Pressure Cooker. Secure the lid and choose the "Poultry" mode. Cook for 15 minutes at High pressure. Once cooking is complete, use a quick pressure release; carefully remove the lid. Add the green beans and secure the lid again; let it sit in the residual heat until wilts. Enjoy!

Easy Spicy Chicken Wings

INGREDIENTS for Servings: 4

3 lbs chicken wings	½ tsp black pepper
2 tbsp olive oil	½ tsp paprika
¼ cup light brown sugar	½ tsp salt
½ tsp garlic powder	1½ cups chicken broth or water
½ tsp cayenne pepper	

DIRECTIONS and Cooking Time: 20 Minutes

Rinse and dry the chicken wings with a paper towel. Put in the large bowl. In a medium bowl, combine the olive oil, sugar, garlic powder, cayenne pepper, black pepper, paprika, and salt. Mix well. Rub all sides of the chicken with the spice mix. Pour the chicken broth into the Electric Pressure Cooker and add the wings. Close and lock the lid. Select the MANUAL setting and set the cooking time for 10 minutes at HIGH pressure. Once pressure cooking is complete, use a Quick Release. Carefully unlock the lid. If you want a crisp skin, slide under the broiler for 5-6 minutes. Serve.

Cheesy Chicken Quinoa

INGREDIENTS for Servings: 2-4

2 tbsp butter	1 tsp dried basil
2 leeks, sliced	Salt and black pepper to taste
3 garlic cloves, minced	1 ½ cups frozen green peas, thawed
1 ½ cups quick-cooking quinoa	1 cup ricotta cheese
1 tbsp chopped rosemary	1 lemon, 2 tbsp zest, and juice
2 ¾ cups chicken broth	¼ cup fresh parsley, chopped
2 chicken breasts, cut into bite-size pieces	1 cup grated Parmesan cheese

DIRECTIONS and Cooking Time: 15 Minutes
Set your Electric Pressure Cooker to Sauté. Melt butter in inner pot and sauté leeks until bright green and softened, 3 minutes. Mix in garlic and sauté until fragrant, 2 minutes. Add quinoa, rosemary, chicken broth, chicken, basil, salt, and black pepper; give ingredients a good stir. Seal the lid, select Manual on High, and set time to 1 minute. Perform a quick pressure release to let out all the steam and unlock lid. Stir in ricotta cheese, green peas, lemon zest, lemon juice, half of parsley, and Parmesan cheese. Press Sauté and continue cooking until cheese melts and chicken cooks through, 6 minutes. Adjust taste with salt and black pepper. Spoon quinoa into serving bowls and garnish with remaining parsley.

Electric Pressure Cooker Chicken Creole

INGREDIENTS for Servings: 6

½ cup butter	½ teaspoon white pepper
4 chicken breasts, boneless	½ teaspoon black pepper
1 cup chopped onion	½ teaspoon cayenne pepper
½ cup chopped celery	½ teaspoon dried basil
½ cup green bell pepper, chopped	1 cup chopped tomatoes
1 teaspoon coconut sugar	1 cup tomato sauce
¼ teaspoon ground cloves	

1 teaspoon garlic powder	1 cup chicken broth Salt to taste

DIRECTIONS and Cooking Time: 15 Minutes
Press the Sauté button on the Electric Pressure Cooker. Heat the butter and stir in the chicken breasts, onion, and celery. Stir until fragrant and the chicken lightly brown.   Add the rest of the ingredients.   Scrape the bottom of the pot to remove the browning.   Close the lid and press the Poultry button.6. Adjust the cooking time to 15 minutes.   Do quick pressure release.

Saucy Chicken Teriyaki

INGREDIENTS for Servings: 8

1 cup chicken broth	¾ cup soy sauce
¾ cup brown sugar	1 ½ lb pineapple, fresh
2 tbsp ground ginger	
Salt and black pepper to taste	2 tbsp garlic powder
3 lb chicken thighs	1 tbsp oregano
	1 tbsp sage

DIRECTIONS and Cooking Time: 25 Minutes
In th IP, stir in all ingredients, except for the chicken. Add the chicken meat and turn to coat. Seal the lid, press Poultry and cook for 20 minutes at High. Do a quick pressure release. Serve.

Turkey With Smoked Paprika

INGREDIENTS for Servings: 5

2 lbs turkey thighs.	¼ cup parsley fresh, chopped
½ cup olive oil	
8 cloves garlic minced	2 tablespoons oregano fresh, chopped
2 tablespoons smoked paprika	
	½ teaspoon salt.½ teaspoon black pepper.
½ teaspoon red pepper flakes	
	½ cup water

DIRECTIONS and Cooking Time: 50 Minutes
Pour the oil into the Electric Pressure Cooker. Select the 'sauté' function.   Add the garlic, smoked paprika, herbs, and red pepper flakes. Cook for 1 minute.   Add the salt and pepper to taste.   Pour this mixture over the turkey thighs, generously coating them.   Add the water to the pot. Place a trivet inside.   Put the coated turkey thighs on the trivet.   Secure the lid. Set the 'manual' function to high pressure for 50 minutes. Once it beeps, release the steam naturally, then remove the lid.   Take out the turkey thighs and slice them.   Sprinkle fresh parsley and oregano and serve.

Asian-style Chicken

INGREDIENTS for Servings: 2

1 tbsp butter	1 pound boneless, skinless chicken legs
½ onion, minced	
⅓ tbsp grated fresh ginger	1 tomato, pureed in a blender

⅓ tbsp minced fresh garlic	2 tbsp chopped fresh cilantro, divided
¼ tsp ground turmeric	⅓ tbsp Indian curry paste
⅓ tbsp kashmiri red chili powder	1 tbsp dried fenugreek
5 oz canned coconut milk, refrigerated overnight	⅓ tsp garam masala
	Salt to taste

DIRECTIONS and Cooking Time: 30 Minutes
Melt butter on Sauté. Add in 1 teaspoon salt and onion. Cook for 2 to 3 minutes until fragrant. Stir in ginger, turmeric, garlic, and red chili powder to coat; cook for 2 more minutes.   Place water and coconut cream into separate bowls. Stir the water from the coconut milk can, pureed tomatoes, and chicken with the onion mixture. Seal lid and cook on High for 8 minutes. Release the Pressure quickly.   Stir coconut cream, fenugreek, curry paste, half the cilantro, and garam masala through the chicken mixture; apply salt for seasoning.   Simmer the mixture and cook for 10 minutes until the sauce thickens, on Sauté. Garnish with the rest of the cilantro before serving.

Peppered Chicken With Chunky Salsa

INGREDIENTS for Servings: 2-4

1 lb chicken breasts	1 onion, sliced
2 tbsp olive oil	Salt and black pepper to taste
3 mixed-colour peppers, cut into strips	
	½ tsp oregano
	½ tsp cumin
2 jalapeño peppers, sliced	2 cups chunky salsa

DIRECTIONS and Cooking Time: 40 Minutes
Warm the olive oil in your Electric Pressure Cooker on Sauté. Place in onion, peppers, and jalapeño peppers and sauté for 5 minutes. Sprinkle chicken breasts with salt and pepper and place in the pot among oregano, cumin, chunky salsa, and ½ cup of water. Seal the lid and cook for 15 minutes on Poultry on High pressure. When ready, perform a quick pressure release and unlock the lid. Shred chicken before serving.

Rosemary Whole Chicken With Asparagus Sauce

INGREDIENTS for Servings: 4

1 (3 ½ lb) young whole chicken	4 fresh thyme, minced
	2 tbsp olive oil
4 garlic cloves, minced	8 oz asparagus, trimmed and chopped
1 tsp olive oil	
3 fresh rosemary, minced	1 onion, chopped
	1 cup chicken stock
2 lemons, zested and quartered	1 tbsp soy sauce
	1 fresh thyme sprig

Salt and black pepper to taste	1 tbsp flour Chopped parsley to garnish

DIRECTIONS and Cooking Time: 40 Minutes
Rub all sides of the chicken with garlic, rosemary, black pepper, lemon zest, thyme, and salt. Into the chicken cavity, insert lemon wedges. Warm oil on Sauté. Add in onion and asparagus, and Sauté for 5 minutes until softened. Mix chicken stock, 1 thyme sprig, black pepper, soy sauce, and salt. Into the inner pot, set trivet over asparagus mixture. On top of the trivet, place the chicken with breast-side up. Seal the lid, select Poultry and cook for 20 minutes on High Pressure. Do a quick release. Remove the chicken to a serving platter. In the inner pot, sprinkle flour over asparagus mixture and blend the sauce with an immersion blender until desired consistency. Top the chicken with asparagus sauce and garnish with parsley.

Sage Chicken With Potatoes & Snow Beans

INGREDIENTS for Servings: 6

2 lb chicken thighs ¼ tsp dried parsley ¼ tsp dried sage Juice of 1 lemon ½ cup chicken broth 1 garlic clove, minced	3 tbsp olive oil 1 lb snow beans 1 lb red potatoes, halved Salt and black pepper to taste

DIRECTIONS and Cooking Time: 25 Minutes
Heat olive oil on Sauté and cook until they sizzling. Add minced garlic and cook for a minute. Place in the thighs and cook them on both sides until golden. Stir in the herbs and the lemon juice and cook for an additional minute until fragrant. Add all remaining ingredients and stir to combine. Seal the lid and cook on Manual at High for 15 minutes. When done, release the pressure quickly. Serve immediately.

Egg And Potato Mayo Salad

INGREDIENTS for Servings: 2-4

1½ cups water 6 russet potatoes, peeled and diced 4 large eggs 1 cup mayonnaise 2 tbsp fresh parsley, chopped	¼ cup onion, chopped 1 tbsp dill pickle juice 1 tbsp mustard Pinch of salt Pinch of ground black pepper

DIRECTIONS and Cooking Time: 20 Minutes
Pour the water into the Electric Pressure Cooker and insert a steamer basket. Place the potatoes and eggs in the basket. Close and lock the lid. Select the MANUAL setting and set the cooking time for 5 minutes at HIGH pressure. Once pressure cooking is complete, use a Quick Release. Carefully unlock the lid. Transfer the eggs to the bowl of cold water and cool for 2-3 minutes. In a medium bowl, combine the mayonnaise, parsley, onion, dill pickle juice, and mustard. Mix well. Add salt and pepper. Peel and slice the eggs. Toss the potatoes and eggs in the bowl. Stir and serve.

Thanksgiving Turkey Breasts

INGREDIENTS for Servings: 6

1/4 cup dry white wine 1 cup turkey stock 2 bell peppers, deseeded and chopped 1/2 teaspoon dried dill 1 serrano pepper, deseeded and chopped 2 garlic cloves, minced	1 teaspoon dried sage 3 tablespoons olive oil 2 thyme sprigs 2 tablespoons butter 1 tablespoon flour 2 ½ pounds turkey breasts Sea salt and ground black pepper, to taste

DIRECTIONS and Cooking Time: 35 Minutes
Add the turkey, peppers, garlic, turkey stock, olive oil, thyme, sage, dried dill, salt, and black pepper to the inner pot. Secure the lid. Choose the "Manual" mode and cook for 25 minutes at High pressure. Once cooking is complete, use a natural pressure release; carefully remove the lid. Press the "Sauté" button again and melt the butter. Now, add the flour, wine, salt, and pepper; let it cook until the sauce has thickened. Spoon the gravy over the turkey breasts and serve warm. Bon appétit!

Classic Lemon Chicken

INGREDIENTS for Servings: 4

4 chicken thighs 2 tbsps. fresh lemon juice 1 medium red onion, sliced	2 tsps. olive oil 1 garlic clove, crushed 1 cup water

DIRECTIONS and Cooking Time: 10 Minutes
Line a baking pan with parchment paper and set aside. In a mixing bowl, thoroughly mix olive oil and lemon juice. Add the chicken thighs and toss to coat. Transfer to the baking pan and top with the garlic and onion slices. Pour 1 cup water into the Electric Pressure Cooker. Arrange a steamer basket inside it and place the baking pan on the basket. Lock the lid. Select the Manual mode and cook for 6 minutes at High Pressure. Once cooking is complete, do a quick pressure release. Carefully open the lid. Allow to cool for 5 minutes before serving.

Fried Turkey Meatballs With Pasta

INGREDIENTS for Servings: 2-4

2 tbsp canola oil 1 pound ground turkey 1 egg ¼ cup bread crumbs 2 cloves garlic, minced 1 tsp dried oregano	Salt and black pepper to taste 3 cups tomato sauce ounces rigatoni 2 tbsp Grana Padano cheese, grated

DIRECTIONS and Cooking Time: 40 Minutes
In a bowl, combine turkey, crumbs, cumin, garlic, and egg. Season with oregano, salt, red pepper flakes, and pepper. Form the mixture into meatballs with well-oiled hands. Warm the oil on Sauté. Cook the meatballs for 3 to 4 minutes, until browned on all sides. Remove to a plate. Add rigatoni to the cooker and cover with tomato sauce. Pour enough water to cover the pasta. Stir well. Throw in the meatballs. Seal the lid and cook for 10 minutes on High Pressure. Release the Pressure quickly. Serve topped with Grana Padano cheese. MEAT recipes

Smoky Paprika Chicken

INGREDIENTS for Servings: 6

2 tbsps. smoked paprika 2 lbs. chicken breasts	Salt and pepper, to taste 1 tbsp. olive oil ½ cup water

DIRECTIONS and Cooking Time: 15 Minutes
Press the Sauté button on the Electric Pressure Cooker and heat the olive oil. Stir in the chicken breasts and smoked paprika and cook for 3 minutes until lightly golden. Season with salt and pepper and add ½ cup water. Lock the lid. Select the Manual mode and cook for 12 minutes at High Pressure. Once cooking is complete, do a natural pressure release for 8 minutes, then release any remaining pressure. Carefully open the lid. Garnish with cilantro or scallions, if desired.

Awesome Chicken In Tikka Masala Sauce

INGREDIENTS for Servings: 4

2 pounds boneless, skinless chicken thighs, Salt and black pepper to taste 1 ½ tbsp olive oil ½ onion, chopped 2 garlic cloves, minced 3 tbsp tomato puree 1 tsp fresh ginger, minced 1 tbsp garam masala 2 tsp curry powder	1 tsp ground coriander ½ tsp ground cumin 1 jalapeño pepper, seeded and chopped 29 ounces canned tomato sauce 3 tomatoes, chopped ½ cup natural yogurt 1 lemon, juiced ¼ cup fresh chopped cilantro leaves 4 lemon wedges

DIRECTIONS and Cooking Time: 40 Minutes

Rub black pepper and ½ teaspoon of salt onto chicken. Warm oil on Sauté. Add garlic and onion and cook for 3 minutes until soft. Stir in tomato puree, garam masala, cumin, curry powder, ginger, coriander, and jalapeño pepper; cook for 30 seconds until fragrant. Stir in remaining ½ teaspoon salt, tomato sauce, and tomatoes. Simmer the mixture as you scrape the bottom to get rid of any browned bits; Stir in chicken to coat. Seal the lid and cook on High Pressure for 10 minutes. Release the Pressure quickly. Press Sauté and simmer the sauce and cook for 3 to 5 minutes until thickened. Stir lemon juice and yogurt through the sauce. Serve garnished with lemon wedges and cilantro.

Sesame Chicken Teriyaki

INGREDIENTS for Servings: 4

1 lb boneless, skinless chicken breasts.½ cup soy sauce1/3 cup honey 2 tablespoons apple cider vinegar. 2 garlic cloves, minced	1 teaspoon sesame oil 2 teaspoons minced ginger 2 tablespoons corn starch 3 tablespoons water Garnish: sliced green onions, sesame seeds

DIRECTIONS and Cooking Time: 10 Minutes
Place the chicken in the pressure cooker pot. In a separate small bowl, mix the soy sauce, sesame oil, ginger, garlic, vinegar and honey. Mix the ingredients well. Pour the prepared mixture over the chicken in the pot. Close the cooker lid and lock it. Select the 'manual' function and set on high pressure for 5 minutes. Let it cook. When the completion beep sounds, use the 'natural release' to vent all the pressure. This should take around 15 minutes. Remove the chicken from the pot and shred it using two forks. Put it to one side. Select the 'sauté function and add the corn-starch and water to the remaining mixture. Cook the sauce while stirring until it thickens. Now add the chicken to the sauce and mix well. Serve it with sprinkled sesame seeds and green onions on top.

Chicken Siciliano With Marsala Wine

INGREDIENTS for Servings: 4

4 chicken drumsticks, boneless 1 teaspoon Italian seasoning mix 2 bell peppers, deseeded and sliced 4 cloves garlic, smashed 1 cup scallions, chopped	1/4 cup Marsala wine 1 cup chicken broth 2 tablespoons butter, room temperature 1/4 cup all-purpose flour 1/4 cup cream cheese Sea salt and ground black pepper, to taste

DIRECTIONS and Cooking Time: 25 Minutes
Press the "Sauté" button to preheat your Electric Pressure Cooker. Melt 1 tablespoon of the butter. Dredge your chicken in the flour; season with spices and cook until slightly brown; reserve. Melt the remaining tablespoon of butter and sauté the peppers, scallions, and garlic. Pour in the wine, scraping up any browned bits from the bottom of the pan. Add the chicken broth and secure the lid. Choose the "Manual" mode and cook for 10 minutes at High pressure. Once cooking is complete, use a natural pressure release; carefully remove the lid. Press the "Sauté" button to preheat your Electric Pressure Cooker one more time. Add the cream cheese and cook for a further 4 to 5 minutes or until everything is thoroughly heated. To serve, spoon the sauce over the chicken drumsticks. Bon appétit!

Shredded Chicken With Marinara

INGREDIENTS for Servings: 4-6

4 lbs chicken breasts	1 tsp salt
½ cup chicken broth	2 cups marinara sauce
½ tsp black pepper	

DIRECTIONS and Cooking Time: 40 Minutes
Add the chicken breasts, broth, pepper, and salt to the Electric Pressure Cooker, stir well. Close and lock the lid. Select MANUAL and cook at HIGH pressure for 20 minutes. Once pressure cooking is complete, use a Quick Release. Unlock and carefully open the lid. Shred the chicken in the pot. Select the SAUTÉ setting. Add the marinara sauce and simmer for 5 minutes. Serve with cooked rice, potato, peas or green salad.

Sage Chicken In Orange Gravy

INGREDIENTS for Servings: 8

1 whole chicken (about 3.5 lb)	3 cups chicken broth
¼ cup oil	1 cup red wine
2 tbsp fresh sage, minced	5 tbsp butter
2 tbsp lemon zest	1 cup orange juice
1 tsp garlic powder	1 tsp sugar
¼ tsp red pepper flakes	½ cup flour
	Salt and black pepper to taste

DIRECTIONS and Cooking Time: 45 Minutes
Mix oil, tarragon, lemon zest, garlic, salt, black pepper, and red pepper. Rub the mixture onto chicken. Melt butter on Sauté. and brown the chicken for 3-4 minutes. Pour in broth and wine. Seal the lid and cook on Poultry for 30 minutes on High. Do a quick release and remove the chicken. In a bowl, mix the orange juice, 1 cup of cooking liquid, flour, and sugar. Cook for 5 minutes on Sauté mode until sauce has thickened. Scatter the sauce over the chicken and serve.

Sticky Sesame Chicken

INGREDIENTS for Servings: 4-6

6 boneless chicken thigh fillets	4 peeled and crushed cloves garlic
5 tbsp sweet chili sauce	1 tbsp rice vinegar
5 tbsp hoisin sauce	1½ tbsp sesame seeds
1 chunk peeled, grated fresh ginger	1 tbsp soy sauce
	½ cup chicken stock

DIRECTIONS and Cooking Time: 35 Minutes
In a medium bowl, whisk together the chili sauce, hoisin sauce, ginger, garlic, vinegar, sesame seeds, soy sauce, and chicken stock until combined. Add the chicken thigh fillets to the Electric Pressure Cooker and pour over the sauce mixture. Close and lock the lid. Select MANUAL and cook at HIGH pressure for 15 minutes. Once cooking is complete, let the pressure Release Naturally for 10 minutes. Release any remaining steam manually. Open the lid. Serve with cooked rice, mashed potato or any other garnish.

Paprika Rosemary Chicken

INGREDIENTS for Servings: 2-4

1 tbsp fresh rosemary leaves	2 tbsp olive oil
6 garlic cloves, minced	4 tbsp balsamic vinegar
Salt and black pepper to taste	1 lemon, zested and juiced
½ tsp smoked paprika	1 cup chicken broth
3 lb whole chicken, cleaned and rinsed	1 large white onion, diced

DIRECTIONS and Cooking Time: 50 Minutes
In a bowl, mix rosemary, garlic, salt, pepper, and paprika. Rub spice mixture all over chicken. Set your Electric Pressure Cooker to Sauté. Heat olive oil in inner pot and sear chicken all around until golden, 7 minutes. Remove to a plate. Pour balsamic vinegar, lemon zest, lemon juice, and chicken broth into the pot. Using a spatula, scrape the stuck bits at the bottom of the pot. Place onion and then chicken in inner pot. Seal the lid, select Manual on High, and set cooking time to 18 minutes. After cooking, perform a natural pressure release for 10 minutes. Remove chicken onto a plate and cover with foil for 5 minutes before slicing. Serve warm.

Whole Chicken With White Wine

INGREDIENTS for Servings: 6

1 (3.5-lb) whole chicken	½ cup chicken broth
1 scallion, minced	1 ½ tbsp olive oil
2 tbsp sugar	1 tbsp celery, chopped
1 tbsp ginger, grated	Salt and black pepper to taste
2 tsp soy sauce	
¼ cup white wine	

DIRECTIONS and Cooking Time: 45 Minutes
Heat oil on Sauté. Season chicken with sugar, salt and pepper, and brown on all sides for a few minutes. Remove from pot and set aside. Stir in wine, broth, soy sauce, celery and scallions. Add chicken and seal the lid. Cook for 35 minutes on Manual at High. When ready, release the pressure quickly.

Green Chili Chicken

INGREDIENTS for Servings: 6

1 ½ lb chicken legs, cut up, bone-in	2 tsp dry basil
Salt and black pepper to taste	½ cup parsley, chopped
For green Chili Sauce:	1 tsp sugar
2 green chili peppers, halved	1 clove garlic, chopped
	2 tbsp lime juice
	¼ cup olive oil

DIRECTIONS and Cooking Time: 25 Minutes
Fit in a trivet and pour in 1 cup of water. Season the chicken with salt, black pepper and basil, and place on the trivet. Seal the lid and cook for 20 minutes at High. When done, release the pressure quickly. Prepare the sauce by mixing all sauce ingredients in a food processor. Blend until well combined. Plate the chicken and top with the sauce.

Tasty Indian Chicken Curry

INGREDIENTS for Servings: 6

2 tbsp butter	2 pounds boneless, skinless chicken legs
1 large onion, minced	3 tomatoes, pureed in a blender
1 tbsp grated fresh ginger	½ cup chopped fresh cilantro, divided
1 tbsp minced fresh garlic	2 tbsp Indian curry paste
½ tsp ground turmeric	2 tbsp dried fenugreek
1 tbsp kashmiri red chili powder	2 tsp sugar
1 (14.5 oz) can coconut milk, refrigerated overnight	1 tsp garam masala
	Salt to taste

DIRECTIONS and Cooking Time: 30 Minutes
Melt butter on Sauté mode. Add in 1 teaspoon salt and onion. Cook for 2 to 3 minutes until fragrant. Stir in ginger, turmeric, garlic, and red chili powder to coat; cook for 2 more minutes. Place water and coconut milk into separate bowls. Stir the water from the coconut milk can, pureed tomatoes, and chicken with the onion mixture. Seal the lid and cook on High Pressure for 8 minutes. Release the Pressure quickly. Stir sugar, coconut milk, fenugreek, curry paste, half the cilantro, and garam masala through the chicken mixture; apply salt for seasoning. Simmer the mixture and cook for 10 minutes until the sauce thickens, on Sauté mode. Garnish with the rest of the cilantro before serving.

Rice & Lentil Chicken With Parsley

INGREDIENTS for Servings: 4

1 tsp olive oil	3 cups chicken broth
1 garlic clove, minced	1 cup white rice
1 small yellow onion, chopped	½ cup dried lentils
4 boneless, skinless chicken thighs	Salt and black pepper to taste
	Chopped fresh parsley for garnish

DIRECTIONS and Cooking Time: 35 Minutes
Warm oil on Sauté mode. Stir-fry onion and garlic for 3 minutes. Add in broth, rice, lentils, chicken, pepper and salt. Seal the lid and cook on High Pressure for 15 minutes. Do a quick release. Remove and shred the chicken in a large bowl. Set the lentils and rice into serving plates, Top with shredded chicken and parsley to serve.

Chicken Marrakesh

INGREDIENTS for Servings: 6

1 onion, sliced	2 carrots, diced
4 tbsp butter	2 cloves garlic, minced
2 lb chicken breasts, cubed	1 tsp parsley, dried
¼ tsp ground cinnamon	Salt and black pepper to taste
½ tsp ground turmeric	1 (14.5-oz) can tomatoes
½ tsp ground cumin	2 cups chicken broth
1 (14-oz) can garbanzo beans	Chopped chives for garnish
2 large sweet potatoes, diced	

DIRECTIONS and Cooking Time: 35 Minutes
Mix cumin, cinnamon, black pepper, parsley, turmeric, and salt in a mixing bowl and stir well to combine. Cut the chicken into cubes and rub with this mixture. Melt the butter on Sauté in the IP and cook the chicken for 5 minutes, stirring occasionally. Add in the remaining ingredients and mix well. Seal the lid, select Manual at High, and cook for 20 minutes. Do a quick release. Serve the dish hot, topped with freshly chopped chives.

Chicken In Garlic-mustard Sauce

INGREDIENTS for Servings: 2

1 lb chicken breasts, boneless and skinless	2 tbsp Dijon mustard
¼ cup apple cider vinegar	¼ tsp black pepper, freshly ground
1 tsp garlic powder	2 tbsp olive oil
	2 cups chicken stock

DIRECTIONS and Cooking Time: 35 Minutes
Season the meat with garlic and black pepper. Place in the Electric Pressure Cooker and Pour in the stock. Seal the lid and cook on Poultry mode for 20 minutes on High. Do a quick release and remove the meat along with the stock. In a bowl, mix olive oil, dijon, and apple cider. Pour into the pot and Press Sauté. Place the meat in this mixture and cook for 10 minutes, turning once. When done, remove from the pot and drizzle with the sauce.

Chicken Salsa
INGREDIENTS for Servings: 2

1 lb frozen, skinless, boneless chicken breast halves	11 oz.) packet taco seasoning mix
½ cup salsa	½ cup chicken broth.

DIRECTIONS and Cooking Time: 15 Minutes
Place the chicken breasts in the Electric Pressure Cooker. Sprinkle taco seasoning uniformly over both sides of the chicken breasts. Add the salsa and chicken broth to the pot. Secure the lid. Set the 'poultry' function on your pressure cooker to cook for 15 minutes. After the beep, release the steam naturally for 20 minutes. Use 'quick release' to vent any remaining steam. Remove the chicken and shred it. Serve the shredded chicken with the steaming hot sauce.

Garlic Chicken
INGREDIENTS for Servings: 4

1 lb chicken breasts	2 garlic cloves, minced
Salt and black pepper to taste	2 tbsp tarragon, chopped
2 tbsp butter	
1 cup chicken broth	

DIRECTIONS and Cooking Time: 25 Minutes
Place chicken breasts in your Electric Pressure Cooker. Sprinkle with garlic, salt, and pepper. Pour in the chicken broth and butter. Seal the lid, select Manual, and cook for 15 minutes on High pressure. When over, allow a natural release for 10 minutes and unlock the lid. Remove the chicken and shred it. Top with tarragon and serve.

Turkey With Garlic Herb Sauce
INGREDIENTS for Servings: 4

4 turkey thighs with skin and bones	2 teaspoons fresh thyme, chopped
Salt and pepper to taste	2 teaspoons fresh oregano, chopped
2 tablespoons olive oil	½ cup sherry, or dry red wine
8 cloves garlic, minced	
½ cup chicken broth	Fresh herbs for topping

DIRECTIONS and Cooking Time: 20 Minutes
Add the salt and pepper seasoning to the turkey thighs. Select the 'sauté' function on the Electric Pressure Cooker, and add the olive oil to it. Place the turkey thighs in the pot and let them cook for 5 minutes on both sides. Remove the turkey thighs when they turn golden brown. Now, put the oil, garlic, thyme and oregano into the pot and 'sauté' for 2 minutes. Add the sherry or wine), chicken broth and fried turkey thighs to the pot. Secure the lid and select the 'manual' function on high pressure for 20 minutes. After the beep, use the 'natural release' to vent the steam. Serve with fresh herbs sprinkled on top.

Turkey Fillets With Cremini Mushrooms
INGREDIENTS for Servings: 6

2 cups Crimini mushrooms, halved or quartered	1 cup water
	2 cloves garlic, peeled and crushed
1/2 teaspoon turmeric powder	1 cup coconut cream
1 ½ pounds turkey fillets	1 teaspoon fresh coriander, minced
A bunch of scallions, chopped	Sea salt and freshly ground black pepper, to taste
1 tablespoon olive oil	1/2 teaspoon brown yellow mustard

DIRECTIONS and Cooking Time: 30 Minutes
Press the "Sauté" button to preheat your Electric Pressure Cooker. Heat the oil and sear the turkey fillets for 2 to 3 minutes per side. Stir in the scallion, mushrooms and garlic; sauté them for 2 minutes more or until they are tender and fragrant. Next, add the salt, black pepper, mustard, turmeric powder, and water to the Electric Pressure Cooker. Secure the lid. Choose the "Meat/Stew" setting and cook for 20 minutes under High pressure. Once cooking is complete, use a quick pressure release; carefully remove the lid. Then, fold in the coconut cream and seal the lid. Let it sit in the residual heat until everything is thoroughly warmed. Garnish with coriander. Bon appétit!

Chicken With Cheese Parsley Dip
INGREDIENTS for Servings: 6

6 chicken drumsticks	1/3 cup cream cheese
1 red chili pepper	1/2 teaspoon cayenne pepper
1/4 cup sesame oil	
2 garlic cloves, minced	1 tablespoon fresh lime juice
Sea salt and ground black pepper, to taste	1/3 cup mayonnaise
1 cup dry white wine	1 garlic clove, minced
Cheese Parsley Dip:	1/2 cup fresh parsley leaves, chopped

DIRECTIONS and Cooking Time: 1 Hour 15 Minutes
Place the garlic, whine, chili pepper, salt, black pepper, and sesame oil in a ceramic container. Add chicken drumsticks; let them marinate for 1 hour in your refrigerator. Add the chicken drumsticks, along with the marinade, to the Electric Pressure Cooker. Secure the lid. Choose the "Poultry" setting and cook for 10 minutes. Once cooking is complete, use a quick pressure release; carefully remove the lid. In a mixing bowl, thoroughly combine parsley, cream cheese mayonnaise, garlic, cayenne pepper, and lime juice. Serve the chicken drumsticks with the parsley sauce on the side. Bon appétit!

Quick Swiss Chard & Chicken Stew

INGREDIENTS for Servings: 4

2 lb chicken breasts, boneless, skinless, cut into pieces	2 tbsp butter, unsalted
	2 tbsp olive oil
	Salt and black pepper to taste
2 lb Swiss chard, chopped	
2 cups chicken broth	

DIRECTIONS and Cooking Time: 30 Minutes
Add the chicken, oil and broth to the pot. Season with salt and black pepper, seal the lid and cook on Manual for 13 minutes on High. Do a quick release, add Swiss chard and butter. Cook on Sauté for 5 minutes. Serve warm.

Creole Chicken With Rice

INGREDIENTS for Servings: 4

2 tbsp olive oil	1 cup chicken broth
1 onion, diced	1 cup white rice, rinsed
3 garlic cloves, minced	
1 lb chicken breasts, sliced	1 bell pepper, chopped
1 (14.5-oz) can tomato sauce	2 tsp creole seasoning
	1 tbsp hot sauce

DIRECTIONS and Cooking Time: 45 Minutes
Warm the olive oil in your Electric Pressure Cooker on Sauté. Place in onion and garlic and cook until fragrant, about 3 minutes. Stir in chicken breasts, bell pepper, hot sauce, and creole seasoning. Cook for 3 more minutes. Mix in chicken broth, tomato sauce, and rice and seal the lid. Select Manual and cook for 20 minutes on High pressure. When ready, allow a natural release for 10 minutes and unlock the lid. Serve warm.

Easy Italian Chicken Stew With Potatoes

INGREDIENTS for Servings: 4

2 lb chicken wings	2 tbsp olive oil
2 potatoes, peeled, cut into chunks	1 tsp smoked paprika, ground
2 fire-roasted tomatoes, peeled, chopped	4 cups chicken broth
	2 tbsp fresh parsley, chopped
1 carrot, peeled, cut into chunks	Salt and black pepper to taste
2 garlic cloves, chopped	1 cup spinach, chopped

DIRECTIONS and Cooking Time: 20 Minutes
Rub the chicken with salt, pepper, and paprika, and place in the pot. Add in all remaining ingredients and seal the lid. Cook on High Pressure for 8 minutes. When ready, do a quick release. Serve hot.

FISH & SEAFOOD RECIPES

Indian Meen Kulambu

INGREDIENTS for Servings: 4

2 tablespoons butter	1 teaspoon ground coriander
6 curry leaves	1/2 teaspoon ground cumin
1 onion, chopped	
2 cloves garlic, crushed	Kosher salt and ground black pepper, to taste
1 (1-inch piece fresh ginger, grated	
1 dried Kashmiri chili, minced	1/2 (14-ounce can coconut milk
1 cup canned tomatoes, crushed	1 pound salmon fillets
1/2 teaspoon turmeric powder	1 tablespoon lemon juice

DIRECTIONS and Cooking Time: 10 Minutes
Press the "Sauté" button and melt the butter. Once hot, cook the curry leaves for about 30 seconds. Stir in the onions, garlic, ginger and Kashmiri chili and cook for 2 minutes more or until they are fragrant. Add the tomatoes, turmeric, coriander, cumin, salt, and black pepper. Continue to sauté for 30 seconds more. Add the coconut milk and salmon. Secure the lid. Choose the "Manual" mode and cook for 2 minutes at Low pressure. Once cooking is complete, use a quick pressure release; carefully remove the lid. Spoon the fish curry into individual bowls. Drizzle lemon juice over the fish curry and serve. Enjoy!

Old Bay Crab

INGREDIENTS for Servings: 5

1 teaspoon Old Bay seasoning	1 ½ pounds crabs
2 cloves garlic, minced	1 lemon, sliced
	1 stick butter

DIRECTIONS and Cooking Time: 15 Minutes
Place 1 cup water and a metal trivet in the bottom of your Electric Pressure Cooker. Lower the crabs onto the trivet. Secure the lid. Choose the "Steam" mode and cook for 3 minutes at Low pressure. Once cooking is complete, use a quick pressure release; carefully remove the lid. Reserve. Press the "Sauté" button and melt butter. Once hot, sauté the garlic and Old Bay seasoning for 2 to 3 minutes or until fragrant and thoroughly heated. Add the cooked crabs and gently stir to combine. Serve with lemon slices. Bon appétit!

Chickpea & Olives Seafood Pot

INGREDIENTS for Servings: 2

⅓ cup scallions, cleaned and chopped	1 cup fish broth
⅓ carrot, chopped	5-6 olives, pitted
⅓ lb shrimp, cleaned and deveined	Sea salt and black pepper, to taste
⅓ cup chickpeas, soaked	¼ tsp Italian seasoning mix

DIRECTIONS and Cooking Time: 25 Minutes
Add all ingredients in your Electric Pressure Cooker. Seal the lid and cook on High Pressure for 12 minutes. Release the pressure naturally, for 10 minutes. Serve warm.

Herby Trout Fillets With Olives

INGREDIENTS for Servings: 6

2 lb trout fillets, skin on	1 tbsp fresh rosemary, chopped
½ cup olive oil	1 tbsp dill sprigs, chopped
¼ cup apple cider vinegar	Sea salt and black pepper to taste
1 red onion, chopped	
1 lemon, chopped	3 cups fish stock
2 garlic cloves, crushed	12 black olives

DIRECTIONS and Cooking Time: 1 Hour 20 Minutes
In a bowl, mix oil, apple cider, onion, garlic, rosemary, dill, sea salt, and pepper. Submerge the fillets into this mixture and refrigerate for 1 hour. Grease the bottom of the pot with 4 tbsp of the marinade and pour in the stock. Add the fish, seal the lid and cook on High pressure for 4 minutes. Do a quick release. Serve with lemon and olives.

Salmon With Parsley-lemon Sauce

INGREDIENTS for Servings: 4

4 salmon fillets	1 tsp chipotle powder
1 tbsp honey	1 tbsp chopped fresh parsley
½ tsp cumin	
1 tbsp olive oil	¼ cup lemon juice
1 small shallot, chopped	Salt and black pepper to taste

DIRECTIONS and Cooking Time: 15 Minutes
Pour 1 cup of water in your IP and fit in a trivet. Place the salmon fillets on top. Seal the lid and cook for 3 minutes on Manual at High. Whisk together the remaining ingredients with 1 tbsp hot water to form a sauce. Once cooking is over, release the pressure quickly, and drizzle the sauce over the salmon. Seal the lid again, and cook for 3 more minutes on Manual at High. Do a quick release and serve hot.

Seafood With Halloumi Cheese And Olives

INGREDIENTS for Servings: 4

1 ½ pounds prawns, cleaned	2 ripe tomatoes, chopped

6 ounces Halloumi cheese, sliced 1 teaspoon dried oregano 1/2 cup Kalamata olives, pitted and sliced Sea salt and ground black pepper, to taste	2 garlic cloves, minced 1/2 teaspoon cayenne pepper, or more taste 2 tablespoons fresh cilantro, chopped 1 tablespoon olive oil 1/2 cup scallions, chopped

DIRECTIONS and Cooking Time: 10 Minutes
Press the "Sauté" button to preheat your Electric Pressure Cooker. Then, heat the oil; sauté the scallions and garlic until tender and fragrant. Add the salt, black pepper, cayenne pepper, oregano, tomatoes, and prawns. Secure the lid. Choose the "Manual" mode and Low pressure; cook for 3 minutes. Once cooking is complete, use a quick pressure release; carefully remove the lid. Ladle into serving bowls; top each serving with cheese, olives and fresh cilantro. Bon appétit!

Cá Kho Tộ (caramelized & Braised Fish)

INGREDIENTS for Servings: 4

4 (7-ounce) sea bass fillets 2 tablespoons fresh chives, chopped Sea salt and white pepper, to taste 2 tablespoons soy sauce Juice of 1/2 lime	1 (1-inch) ginger root, grated 1 cup chicken broth 1/4 cup brown sugar 2 tablespoons coconut oil, melted 2 tablespoons fish sauce

DIRECTIONS and Cooking Time: 10 Minutes
Press the "Sauté" button and heat the coconut oil. Once hot, cook the brown sugar, fish sauce, soy sauce, ginger, lime, salt, white pepper, and broth. Bring to a simmer and press the "Cancel" button. Add the sea bass. Secure the lid. Choose the "Manual" mode and cook for 4 minutes at High pressure. Once cooking is complete, use a quick pressure release; carefully remove the lid. Remove the sea bass fillets from the cooking liquid. Press the "Sauté" button one more time. Reduce the sauce until it is thick and syrupy. Spoon the sauce over the reserved sea bass fillets. Garnish with fresh chives. Bon appétit!

Coconut Cod Curry

INGREDIENTS for Servings: 6

2 tablespoons red curry paste 2 teaspoons fish sauce 2 teaspoons honey4 teaspoons Sriracha* 4 cloves garlic, minced 2 teaspoons ground turmeric 2 teaspoons ground ginger	1 28 oz.) can coconut milkJuice of 2 lemons 1 teaspoon sea salt 1 teaspoon white pepper 2 lbs. codfish, cut into 1" cubes 1/2 cup chopped fresh cilantro Garnish4 lime wedges Garnish

DIRECTIONS and Cooking Time: 3 Minutes
Add all the ingredients, except the cod cubes and garnish, to a large bowl and whisk them well. Arrange the cod cube at the base of the Electric Pressure Cooker and pour the coconut milk mixture over it. Secure the lid and hit the "Manual" key, select high pressure with 3 minutes cooking time. After the beep, do a 'Quick release' then remove the lid. Garnish with fresh cilantro and lemon wedges then serve.

Cheesy Tuna

INGREDIENTS for Servings: 4

1 lb tuna fillets 2 tbsp butter Salt and black pepper to taste	1 tbsp flour ½ cup milk 1 cup mozzarella cheese, grated

DIRECTIONS and Cooking Time: 20 Minutes
Melt the butter in your Electric Pressure Cooker on Sauté. Place in flour, salt, and pepper and cook for 1 minute. Pour in milk and cook for 3-5 minutes, stirring often. Stir in mozzarella cheese. Place the tuna fillets in a greased baking pan and pour the cheese sauce over the fish; cover with foil. Clean the pot and add in 1 cup of water. Fit in a trivet. Place the pan on the trivet and seal the lid. Select Manual and cook for 5 minutes on High pressure. When ready, perform a quick pressure release and unlock the lid. Serve warm.

Cod Meal

INGREDIENTS for Servings: 2

1 cup water 1 fresh large fillet cod	2 tbsps. ghee Salt and pepper, to taste

DIRECTIONS and Cooking Time: 5 Minutes
Cut fillet into 3 pieces. Coat with the ghee and season with salt and pepper. Pour the water into the pot and place steamer basket/trivet inside. Arrange the fish pieces over the basket/trivet. Lock the lid. Select the Manual mode and cook for 5 minutes at Low Pressure. Once cooking is complete, do a quick pressure release. Carefully open the lid. Serve warm.

Old Bay Fish Tacos

INGREDIENTS for Servings: 4

2 large cod fillets 1 tablespoon old bay seasoning	1/2 cup quesadilla cheese

DIRECTIONS and Cooking Time: 8 Minutes

Place a trivet or a steamer basket in the Electric Pressure Cooker. Pour a cup of water. Season the cod fillets with old bay seasoning. Place on top of the steamer rack. Close the lid and press the Steam button. Adjust the cooking time to 10 minutes. Do quick pressure release. Serve with quesadilla cheese on top.

Mahi-mahi With Tomatoes

INGREDIENTS for Servings: 3

3 4 oz.) mahi-mahi fillets1 ½ tablespoons butter	½ teaspoon dried oregano
½ yellow onion, sliced	1 tablespoon fresh lemon juice
Salt and freshly ground black pepper, to taste	1 14 oz.) can sugar-free diced tomatoes

DIRECTIONS and Cooking Time: 14 Minutes
Add the butter to the Electric Pressure Cooker. Select the "Sauté" function on it. Add all the ingredient to the pot except the fillets. Cook them for 10 minutes. Press the "Cancel" key, then add the mahi-mahi fillets to the sauce. Cover the fillets with sauce by using a spoon. Secure the lid and set the "Manual" function at high pressure for 4 minutes. After the beep, do a Quick release then remove the lid. Serve the fillets with their sauce, poured on top.

American Clam Chowder

INGREDIENTS for Servings: 2

2 pieces of bacon, chopped	1 tablespoon flour
½ tablespoon olive oil	¼ cup chopped celery
½ onion, chopped	1 teaspoon nutmeg
½ clove minced garlic	1 ½ tablespoons parsley
¼ cup green pepper, chopped	1 8 oz.) can tomatoes, smashed1 ½ cups clam juice
1 medium potatoes, peeled and diced	1 bay leaf
	½ cup minced clam

DIRECTIONS and Cooking Time: 7 Minutes
Add the oil and then bacon to the Electric Pressure Cooker and cook on the "Sauté" settings until it gets crispy. Now add the onion, green pepper, and garlic to the pot. Cook for 3 minutes. Add the clam juice, tomatoes, potatoes, celery, parsley, bay leaf, flour, salt, pepper, and nutmeg in the pot and stir well. Secure the lid and select the "Manual" function for 5 minutes with high pressure. After the beep, do a Quick release then remove the lid. Remove the bay leaf from the mixture and add the clams into it. Let it stay for 5 minutes and then serve hot.

Salmon With Pecan Coating

INGREDIENTS for Servings: 2-4

2 salmon fillets	1 egg, beaten
½ cup olive oil	¼ cup pecans, finely chopped
½ tsp salt	
¼ cup flour	1 cup water

DIRECTIONS and Cooking Time: 25 Minutes
Preheat the Electric Pressure Cooker by selecting SAUTÉ. Add and heat the oil. Season the fillets with salt. Dip the fillets in the flour, then in whisked egg, then in pecans. Add to the pot and brown the fish on both sides. Press the CANCEL button to stop the SAUTE function. Remove the salmon from the pot and place the steam rack in it. Pour in the water. Place the fillets on the steam rack. Close and lock the lid. Select the MANUAL setting and set the cooking time for 4 minutes at HIGH pressure. When the timer beeps, use a Natural Release for 10 minutes. Uncover the pot. Serve.

Fish Packs

INGREDIENTS for Servings: 2

2 tilapia fillets	1 tsp chopped rosemary
2 tbsp olive oil	
2 garlic cloves, minced	Salt and black pepper to taste
2 tomatoes, chopped	
	¼ cup white wine

DIRECTIONS and Cooking Time: 15 Minutes
Cut out 2 heavy-duty foil papers to contain each tilapia. Place each fish on each foil and arrange on top olive oil, garlic, tomatoes, rosemary, salt, black pepper, and drizzle with white wine. Wrap foil tightly to secure fish well. Pour 1 cup of water in inner pot, fit in a trivet with slings, and lay fish packs on top. Seal the lid, select Manual/Pressure Cook mode on High, and set cooking time to 3 minutes. When done cooking, perform a quick pressure release to let out steam, and carefully remove fish packs using tongs. Place on serving plates and open. Serve.

Steamed Mussels In Scallion Sauce

INGREDIENTS for Servings: 4

1 cup water	2 garlic cloves, sliced
1/2 cup cooking wine	2 tablespoons butter
1 ½ pounds frozen mussels, cleaned and debearded	1 bunch scallion, chopped

DIRECTIONS and Cooking Time: 10 Minutes
Add the water, wine, and garlic to the inner pot. Add a metal rack to the inner pot. Put the mussels into the steamer basket; lower the steamer basket onto the rack. Secure the lid. Choose the "Steam" mode and cook for 3 minutes at Low pressure. Once cooking is complete, use a quick pressure release; carefully remove the lid. Press the "Sauté" button and add butter and scallions; let it cook until the sauce is

thoroughly heated and slightly thickened. Press the "Cancel" button and add the mussels. Serve warm. Bon appétit!

Simple Steamed Salmon Fillets

INGREDIENTS for Servings: 3

1 cup water	Salt and pepper, to taste
2 tbsps. freshly squeezed lemon juice	1 tsp. toasted sesame seeds
2 tbsps. soy sauce	
10 oz. salmon fillets	

DIRECTIONS and Cooking Time: 10 Minutes
Set a trivet in the Electric Pressure Cooker and pour the water into the pot. Using a heat-proof dish, combine all ingredients. Place the heat-proof dish on the trivet. Lock the lid. Select the Manual mode and cook for 10 minutes at Low Pressure. Once cooking is complete, do a quick pressure release. Carefully open the lid. Garnish with toasted sesame seeds and serve.

Brussels Sprout Shrimp

INGREDIENTS for Servings: 2

¼ lb large shrimp, cleaned, rinsed	Sea salt and black pepper to taste
2 oz Brussels sprouts, outer leaves removed	¼ cup olive oil, plus ½ tbsp
1 oz whole okra	2 tbsp balsamic vinegar
2 carrots, chopped	½ tbsp fresh rosemary, chopped
¼ cups chicken broth	
½ tomatoes, diced	¼ small celery stalk, for decoration
½ tbsp tomato paste	
1/8 tsp cayenne pepper, ground	½ tbsp sour cream, optionally

DIRECTIONS and Cooking Time: 45 Minutes
Mix 1/4 cup of oil, vinegar, rosemary, salt, and pepper in a large bowl. Stir and submerge the shrimp into the mixture. Toss well to coat and refrigerate for 20 minutes. Add tomatoes, paste, ½ tbsp olive oil, and cayenne pepper. Cook on Sauté for 5 minutes, stirring constantly. Remove to a bowl, cover and set aside. Pour in broth, and add Brussels sprouts, carrots, and okra. Sprinkle with salt, black pepper and seal the lid. Cook on High pressure for 15 minutes. Then, do a quick release. Remove the vegetables and add shrimp in the remaining broth. Seal the lid again and cook on Steam for 3 minutes on High. Do a quick release and set aside. Add the remaining oil, and cooked vegetables. Cook for 2-3 minutes, stirring constantly, on Sauté. Remove to a bowl. Top with sour cream and drizzle with shrimp marinade.

Mediterranean Cod With Cherry Tomatoes

INGREDIENTS for Servings: 4

1 lb cherry tomatoes, halved	Salt and black pepper to taste
1 bunch fresh thyme sprigs	2 cups water
	1 cup white rice
4 fillets cod	1 cup kalamata olives
1 tsp olive oil	2 tbsp pickled capers
1 clove garlic, pressed	1 tbsp olive oil

DIRECTIONS and Cooking Time: 20 Minutes
Line a parchment paper on the basket of the pot. Place about half the tomatoes in a single layer on the paper. Sprinkle with thyme, reserving some for garnish. Arrange cod fillets on top. Sprinkle with olive oil. Spread the garlic, pepper, salt, and remaining tomatoes over the fish. In the pot, mix rice and water. Lay a trivet over the rice and water. Lower steamer basket onto the trivet. Seal the lid, and cook for 7 minutes on Low Pressure. Release the Pressure quickly. Remove the steamer basket and trivet from the pot. Use a fork to fluff rice. Plate the fish fillets and apply a garnish of olives, reserved thyme, remaining olive oil, and capers. Serve with rice.

Delicious Cod With Cherry Tomatoes

INGREDIENTS for Servings: 3

1 lb black cod fillets	¼ cup olive oil
1 tbsp tomato paste	¼ tsp allspice
1 tsp honey	1 garlic clove, minced
1 fresno chili pepper, minced	1 tbsp red wine vinegar
¼ bunch of cilantro, chopped	1 tsp paprika
2 cups cherry tomatoes, halved	½ tsp red pepper flakes

DIRECTIONS and Cooking Time: 20 Minutes
Add the tomato paste, chili pepper, honey, olive oil, allspice, garlic, paprika, and red pepper flakes in a bowl and mix well. Place the fish into the IP, and pour mixture over the fish. Put cherry tomatoes on top of the fish. Add in 1 cup of water. Seal the lid, select Manual at High, and cook for 5 minutes. When ready, perform a natural pressure release for 10 minutes. Serve hot sprinkled with cilantro.

Basil Salmon With Artichokes & Potatoes

INGREDIENTS for Servings: 4

4 salmon fillets	2 tbsp butter
1 lb new potatoes	Salt and black pepper

1 cup artichoke hearts, halved	to taste 2 tbsp basil, chopped

DIRECTIONS and Cooking Time: 30 Minutes
Season the potatoes with salt and pepper. Pour 1 cup of water in your Electric Pressure Cooker and fit in a trivet. Place the potatoes on the trivet and seal the lid. Select Manual and cook for 2 minutes on High pressure. Once over, perform a quick pressure release and unlock the lid. Sprinkle the salmon and artichokes with salt and pepper. Put them on the trivet with the potatoes, sprinkle with basil, and seal the lid. Select Manual and cook for another 5 minutes on High pressure. Once done, allow a natural release for 10 minutes and unlock the lid. Remove potatoes to a bowl and stir in butter until well coated. Serve the salmon with artichokes and potatoes.

Electric Pressure Cooker Mediterranean Fish

INGREDIENTS for Servings: 3

¼ cup red wine 1 tablespoon red wine vinegar 1 tablespoon lemon juice, freshly squeezed 1 clove of garlic, minced	¼ teaspoon dried oregano 1-pound salmon fillets, fresh 2 sprigs rosemary Salt and pepper 1 tablespoon feta cheese, crumbled

DIRECTIONS and Cooking Time: 6 Minutes
Place all ingredients in the Electric Pressure Cooker except for the feta cheese. Close the lid and press the Manual button. Adjust the cooking time to 6 minutes. Do natural pressure release. Once the lid is open, garnish with feta cheese on top.

Shrimp And Beans Mix

INGREDIENTS for Servings: 3

1 ½ tablespoons olive oil 1 medium onion, chopped ½ celery stalk, chopped 1 garlic clove, minced 1 tablespoon fresh parsley, chopped ½ teaspoon red pepper flakes, crushed	½ small green bell pepper, seeded and chopped ½ teaspoon cayenne pepper ½ lb. great northern beans, rinsed, soaked, and drained 1 cup chicken broth 1 bay leaf ½ lb. medium shrimp, peeled and deveined

DIRECTIONS and Cooking Time: 25 Minutes
Select the "Sauté" function on your Electric Pressure Cooker, then add the oil, onion, celery, bell pepper and cook for 5 minutes. Now add the parsley, garlic, spices, and bay leaf to the pot and cook for another 2 minutes. Pour in the chicken broth then add the beans to it. Secure the cooker lid. Select the "Manual" function for 15 minutes with medium pressure. After the beep, do a Natural release for 10 minutes and remove the lid. Add the shrimp to the beans and cook them together on the "Manual" function for 2 minutes at high pressure. Do a 'Quick release', keep it aside for 10 minutes, then remove the lid. Serve hot.

Extraordinary Greek-style Fish

INGREDIENTS for Servings: 4

2 tablespoons olive oil 1 ½ pounds cod fillets 1 pound tomatoes, chopped Sea salt and ground black pepper, to taste	2 sprigs rosemary, chopped 2 sprigs thyme, chopped 1 bay leaf 2 cloves garlic, smashed 1/2 cup Greek olives, pitted and sliced

DIRECTIONS and Cooking Time: 10 Minutes
Place 1 cup of water and a metal trivet in the bottom of the inner pot. Brush the sides and bottom of a casserole dish with olive oil. Place the cod fillets in the greased casserole dish. Add the tomatoes, salt, pepper, rosemary, thyme, bay leaf, and garlic. Lower the dish onto the trivet. Secure the lid. Choose the "Steam" mode and cook for 3 minutes at Low pressure. Once cooking is complete, use a quick pressure release; carefully remove the lid. Serve garnished with Greek olives and enjoy!

Halibut With Cheese-mayo Sauce

INGREDIENTS for Servings: 6

1 ½ pounds halibut steaks 1 teaspoon stone-ground mustard 4 tablespoons cream cheese 2 cloves garlic, minced 1/2 teaspoon salt flakes 2 tablespoons olive oil	Sea salt and ground pepper, to your liking 1 cup wild rice, rinsed and drained 1 tablespoon butter 4 tablespoons mayonnaise 1/2 teaspoon red pepper flakes, crushed

DIRECTIONS and Cooking Time: 1 Hour
In a saucepan, bring 3 cups of water and rice to a boil. Reduce the heat to simmer; cover and let it simmer for 45 to 55 minutes. Add the butter, salt, and red pepper; fluff with a fork. Cover and reserve, keeping your rice warm. Cut 4 sheets of aluminum foil. Place the halibut steak in each sheet of foil. Add the olive oil, salt, and black pepper to the top of the fish; close each packet and seal the edges. Add 1 cup of water and a steamer rack to the bottom of your Electric Pressure Cooker. Lower the packets onto the rack. Secure the lid. Choose the "Steam" mode and cook for 3 minutes

at Low pressure. Once cooking is complete, use a natural pressure release; carefully remove the lid. Meanwhile, mix the cream cheese, mayonnaise, stone-ground mustard, and garlic until well combined. Serve the steamed fish with the mayo sauce and wild rice on the side. Bon appétit!

Mediterranean Cod With Olives

INGREDIENTS for Servings: 2-4

1 lb cherry tomatoes, halved	3 pinches salt
1 bunch fresh thyme sprigs	2 cups water
	1 cup white rice
4 fillets cod	1 cup kalamata olives
1 tsp olive oil	2 tbsp pickled capers
1 clove garlic, pressed	1 tbsp olive oil
	A pinch of ground black pepper

DIRECTIONS and Cooking Time: 20 Minutes
Line a parchment paper on the basket of your Electric Pressure Cooker. Place about half the tomatoes in a single layer on the paper. Sprinkle with thyme, reserving some for garnish. Arrange cod fillets on top. Sprinkle with a little bit of olive oil. Spread the garlic, pepper, salt, and remaining tomatoes over the fish. In the pot, mix rice and water. Lay a trivet over the rice and water. Lower steamer basket onto the trivet. Seal the lid, and cook for 7 minutes on Low Pressure. Release the Pressure quickly. Remove the steamer basket and trivet from the pot. Use a fork to fluff rice. Plate the fish fillets and apply a garnish of olives, reserved thyme, pepper, remaining olive oil, and capers. Serve with rice.

Haddock Fillets With Steamed Green Beans

INGREDIENTS for Servings: 4

1 lime, cut into wedges	4 teaspoons ghee
1/2 cup water	Sea salt and ground black pepper, to taste
4 haddock fillets	2 cloves garlic, minced
1 rosemary sprig	4 cups green beans
2 thyme sprigs	
1 tablespoon fresh parsley	

DIRECTIONS and Cooking Time: 15 Minutes
Place the lime wedges and water in the inner pot. Add a steamer rack. Lower the haddock fillets onto the rack; place the rosemary, thyme, parsley, and ghee on the haddock fillets. Season with salt and pepper. Secure the lid. Choose the "Steam" mode and cook for 3 minutes at Low pressure. Once cooking is complete, use a quick pressure release; carefully remove the lid. Reserve. Then, add the garlic and green beans to the inner pot. Secure the lid. Choose the "Steam" mode and cook for 3 minutes at Low pressure. Once cooking is complete, use a quick pressure release; carefully remove the lid. Serve the haddock fillets with green beans on the side. Bon appétit!

White Wine Oysters

INGREDIENTS for Servings: 6

2 lb in-shell oysters, cleaned	1 garlic clove, minced
1 cup vegetable broth	Salt and black pepper to taste
4 tbsp white wine	4 tbsp butter, melted
2 tbsp thyme, chopped	

DIRECTIONS and Cooking Time: 15 Minutes
Place the vegetable broth, oysters, white wine, garlic, salt, and pepper in your Electric Pressure Cooker and seal the lid. Select Manual and cook for 3 minutes on High pressure. Once done, perform a quick pressure release and unlock the lid. Drain the oysters, drizzle with the melted butter, and top with thyme to serve.

Mustardy Steamed Catfish Fillets

INGREDIENTS for Servings: 2

3/4 lb catfish fillet	1 lemon, juiced
½ cup parsley leaves, chopped	½ tbsp fresh rosemary
	1 ½ cups white wine
2 garlic cloves, crushed	1 ½ tbsp Dijon mustard
½ onion, finely chopped	3/4 cup extra virgin olive oil
½ tbsp fresh dill, chopped	2 cups fish stock

DIRECTIONS and Cooking Time: 50 Minutes
In a bowl, mix lemon juice, parsley, garlic, onion, fresh dill, rosemary, wine, mustard, and oil. Stir well to combine. Submerge fillets in this mixture and cover with a tight lid. Refrigerate for 1 hour. Insert the trivet, remove the fish from the fridge and place it on the rack. Pour in stock along with the marinade and seal the lid. Cook on Steam for 8 minutes on High. Release the pressure quickly and serve.

Clam & Prawn Paella

INGREDIENTS for Servings: 2-4

2 tbsp olive oil	1 tsp turmeric powder
1 onion, chopped	½ tsp salt
4 garlic cloves, minced	1 pound small clams, scrubbed
½ cup dry white wine	
2 cups bomba (Spanish) rice	1 lb fresh prawns, peeled and deveined
4 cups chicken stock	1 red bell pepper, diced
1 ½ tsp sweet paprika	
½ tsp ground black pepper	1 lemon, cut in wedges

DIRECTIONS and Cooking Time: 30 Minutes
Stir-fry onion and garlic in a tbsp of oil on Sauté mode for 3 minutes. Pour in wine to deglaze, scraping the

bottom of the pot of any brown. Cook for 2 minutes, until the wine is reduced by half. Add in rice and water. Season with the paprika, turmeric, salt, and pepper. Seal the lid and cook on High Pressure for 10 minutes. Do a quick release. Remove to a plate and wipe the pot clean. Heat the remaining oil on Sauté. Cook clams and prawns for 6 minutes, until the clams have opened and the shrimp are pink. Discard unopened clams. Arrange seafood and lemon wedges over paella, to serve.

Tunisian-style Couscous

INGREDIENTS for Servings: 4

2 cups couscous	1 teaspoon coriander
2 tablespoons almonds, slivered	1 teaspoon garam masala
1 teaspoon ancho chili powder	1 yellow onion, chopped
1 cup vegetable broth	2 cups water
1 cup coconut milk	2 tablespoons butter
1 teaspoon dried basil	Sea salt and ground black pepper, to taste
2 bay leaves	
4 cardamom pods	1 teaspoon cayenne pepper
2 ripe tomatoes, pureed	1 teaspoon curry paste
1 ½ pounds halibut, cut into chunks	

DIRECTIONS and Cooking Time: 10 Minutes
Press the "Sauté" button and melt the butter. Once hot, cook the onions until tender and translucent. Add the remaining ingredients, except for the slivered almonds, to the inner pot; stir to combine. Secure the lid. Choose the "Manual" mode and cook for 4 minutes at High pressure. Once cooking is complete, use a quick pressure release; carefully remove the lid. Serve garnished with almonds. Bon appétit!

Canned Tuna Casserole

INGREDIENTS for Servings: 4

2 cans (5-oz) tuna, flaked	Salt and black pepper to taste
1 cup celery, diced	1 cup green peas
½ cup mayonnaise	1 ½ cups potato chips, crushed
4 chopped hard-boiled eggs	

DIRECTIONS and Cooking Time: 29 Minutes
Pour 1 cup of water in the IP and insert a trivet. In a bowl, whisk together tuna, celery, mayonnaise, eggs, salt, green peas, and pepper until combined. Pour the mixture into a greased baking dish. Top with crushed potato chips. Place the dish on the trivet. Seal the lid, select Manual at High, and cook for 4 minutes. When ready, do a quick release. Serve warm.

Steamed Halibut Packets

INGREDIENTS for Servings: 4

4 halibut fillets	1 garlic clove, minced
1 lb cherry tomatoes cut into halves	½ tsp thyme
1 cup olives, pitted and chopped	Salt and black pepper to taste
2 tbsp olive oil	Arugula for garnish

DIRECTIONS and Cooking Time: 30 Minutes
Pour 1 cup of water in your Electric Pressure Cooker and insert a trivet. divide the halibut fillets, cherry tomatoes, and olives between 4 sheets of aluminum foil. Drizzle with olive oil and season with salt, pepper, garlic, and thyme. Close the packets and seal the edges. Place them on the trivet. Secure the lid, select Steam, and cook for 4 minutes on Low. When done, allow a natural release for 10 minutes and unlock the lid. Serve scattered with some arugula and enjoy!

Seafood Platter

INGREDIENTS for Servings: 4

1 ½ tablespoons Cajun's shrimp boil½ lb. clams, fresh frozen½ lb. shell on shrimp, deveined½ lb. mussels, fresh or frozen1 lemon, quartered½ lb. smoked Kielbasa, cut into 2-inch pieces	½ lb. medium-sized red potatoes, halved
	1 cup seafood stock
	1 tablespoon chopped parsley
	Cilantro and lemon wedges Garnish

DIRECTIONS and Cooking Time: 40 Minutes
Add the seafood stock, boiling spice, and potatoes to the Electric Pressure Cooker. Cover the lid and let it "Slow Cook" for 30 minutes till the potatoes get tender. Remove the lid and add the clams, shrimp, mussels, Kielbasa, and lemon to the pot. Cook for 10 minutes if you are using frozen seafood, else cook for only 5 minutes. Garnish with cilantro and lemon wedges on top. Serve.

Vietnamese-style Caramel Fish

INGREDIENTS for Servings: 4

2 tablespoons coconut oil, melted	Juice of 1/2 lime
1/4 cup brown sugar	Sea salt and white pepper, to taste
2 tablespoons fish sauce	1 cup chicken broth
2 tablespoons soy sauce	4 (7-ounce sea bass fillets
1 (1-inch ginger root, grated	2 tablespoons fresh chives, chopped

DIRECTIONS and Cooking Time: 10 Minutes
Press the "Sauté" button and heat the coconut oil. Once hot, cook the brown sugar, fish sauce, soy sauce, ginger, lime, salt, white pepper, and broth. Bring to a simmer and press the "Cancel" button. Add sea bass.

93

Secure the lid. Choose the "Manual" mode and cook for 4 minutes at High pressure. Once cooking is complete, use a quick pressure release; carefully remove the lid. Remove the sea bass fillets from the cooking liquid. Press the "Sauté" button one more time. Reduce the sauce until it is thick and syrupy. Spoon the sauce over the reserved sea bass fillets. Garnish with fresh chives. Bon appétit!

Electric Pressure Cooker Lobster Roll

INGREDIENTS for Servings: 6

1 ½ cups chicken broth	1 lemon, halved
1 teaspoon old bay seasoning	3 scallions, chopped
	½ cup mayonnaise
2 pounds lobster tails, raw and in the shell	4 tablespoons unsalted butter
	¼ teaspoon celery salt

DIRECTIONS and Cooking Time: 6 Minutes
Pour the broth into the Electric Pressure Cooker and sprinkle with old bay seasoning. Place a steamer on top and lay each lobster tail shell side down.3. Squeeze the first half of the lemon over the lobsters. Close the lid and press the Manual button. Adjust the cooking time to 6 minutes. While cooking, prepare the sauce by combining the rest of the ingredients in a bowl. Once the timer beeps off, do quick pressure release. Brush the mayo dip on the exposed meat of the lobster tails.

Codfish And Tomato Casserole

INGREDIENTS for Servings: 4

1 ½ pounds cod fillets	1 bay leaf
1/2 cup Greek olives, pitted and sliced	2 cloves garlic, smashed
Sea salt and ground black pepper, to taste	1 pound tomatoes, chopped
2 sprigs rosemary, chopped	2 tablespoons olive oil
	2 sprigs thyme, chopped

DIRECTIONS and Cooking Time: 10 Minutes
Place 1 cup of water and a metal trivet in the bottom of the inner pot. Brush the sides and bottom of a casserole dish with olive oil. Place the cod fillets in the greased casserole dish. Add the tomatoes, salt, pepper, rosemary, thyme, bay leaf, and garlic. Lower the dish onto the trivet. Secure the lid. Choose the "Steam" mode and cook for 3 minutes at Low pressure. Once cooking is complete, use a quick pressure release; carefully remove the lid. Serve garnished with Greek olives and enjoy!

Spicy Haddock Curry

INGREDIENTS for Servings: 4

1 pound haddock	1 teaspoon ground cumin
Sea salt and freshly ground black pepper	1 cup chicken stock
1 can reduced fat coconut milk	2 long red chilis, deseeded and minced
1 onion, chopped	2 tablespoons tamarind paste
2 garlic cloves, minced	2 tablespoons peanut oil
1 teaspoon mustard seeds	
1 teaspoon turmeric powder	1 (1-inch) piece fresh root ginger, peeled and grated

DIRECTIONS and Cooking Time: 10 Minutes
Press the "Sauté" button and heat the peanut oil; once hot, sauté the onion, garlic, ginger, and chilis until aromatic. Add the remaining ingredients and gently stir to combine. Secure the lid. Choose the "Manual" mode and cook for 4 minutes at Low pressure. Once cooking is complete, use a quick pressure release; carefully remove the lid. Divide between serving bowls and serve warm. Enjoy!

Chili-lime Shrimps

INGREDIENTS for Servings: 4

1½ lbs. peeled and deveined raw shrimp	1 tbsp. chili powder
	1 tbsp. coconut oil
Salt and pepper, to taste	2 tbsps. freshly squeezed lime juice

DIRECTIONS and Cooking Time: 4 Minutes
Place all ingredients in the Electric Pressure Cooker. Lock the lid. Select the Manual mode and cook for 4 minutes at Low Pressure. Once cooking is complete, do a quick pressure release. Carefully open the lid. Serve warm.

Orange-butter Sea Bass

INGREDIENTS for Servings: 2

1 tbsp. safflower oil	1 tbsp. tamari sauce
½ lb. sea bass	1 clove garlic, minced
Sea salt, to taste	1 tbsp. melted butter
¼ tsp. white pepper	½ tsp. dried dill weed
1 cup water	
½ orange, juiced	

DIRECTIONS and Cooking Time: 18 Minutes
Press the Sauté button on the Electric Pressure Cooker and heat the safflower oil. Sear the sea bass for about 2 minutes on each side. Sprinkle the salt and white pepper to season. Add the water and steamer rack to the Electric Pressure Cooker, then transfer the sea bass to the steamer rack. Lock the lid. Select the Steam mode and cook for 10 minutes at Low Pressure. Once cooking is complete, do a quick pressure release. Carefully open the lid. Transfer the sea bass to a plate and set aside. Add the orange juice, tamari sauce, garlic, butter, and dill weed to the cooking liquid in the

Electric Pressure Cooker, and stir to incorporate. Press the Sauté button again and allow to simmer, or until the sauce is thickened. Spoon the sauce over the sea bass and serve warm.

Spicy Thai Prawns

INGREDIENTS for Servings: 4

2 tablespoons coconut oil	1 cup coconut milk
1 small white onion, chopped	2 tablespoons lime juice
2 cloves garlic, minced	1 tablespoon sugar
1 ½ pounds prawns, deveined	Kosher salt and white pepper, to your liking
1/2 teaspoon red chili flakes	1/2 teaspoon cayenne pepper
1 bell pepper, seeded and sliced	1 teaspoon fresh ginger, ground
2 tablespoons fish sauce	2 tablespoons fresh cilantro, roughly chopped

DIRECTIONS and Cooking Time: 10 Minutes
Press the "Sauté" button and heat the coconut oil; once hot, sauté the onion and garlic until aromatic. Add the prawns, red chili flakes, bell pepper, coconut milk, fish sauce, lime juice, sugar, salt, white pepper, cayenne pepper, and ginger. Secure the lid. Choose the "Manual" mode and cook for 3 minutes at Low pressure. Once cooking is complete, use a quick pressure release; carefully remove the lid. Divide between serving bowls and serve garnished with fresh cilantro. Enjoy!

Collard Greens Octopus & Shrimp

INGREDIENTS for Servings: 2-4

1 lb collard greens, chopped	1 lb shrimp, whole
6 oz octopus, cut into bite-sized pieces	3 cups fish stock
	4 tbsp olive oil
1 large tomato, peeled, chopped	3 garlic cloves
	2 tbsp fresh parsley, chopped
	1 tsp sea salt

DIRECTIONS and Cooking Time: 35 Minutes
Place shrimp and octopus in the pot. Add tomato and fish stock. Seal the lid and cook on High Pressure for 15 minutes. Do a quick release. Remove shrimp and octopus, drain the liquid. Heat olive oil on Sauté and add garlic, parsley, and stir-fry until translucent. Add collard greens and simmer for 10 minutes. Season with salt, stir and remove from the cooker. Serve with shrimp and octopus.

Citrus Marinated Smelt With Okra & Cherry Tomatoes

INGREDIENTS for Servings: 4

1 lb fresh smelt, cleaned, heads removed	2 garlic cloves, crushed
1 cup extra virgin olive oil	1 tsp sea salt
	5 oz okra
½ cup freshly squeezed lemon juice	1 carrot, chopped
	¼ cup green peas, soaked overnight
¼ cup freshly squeezed orange juice	5 oz cherry tomatoes, halved
1 tbsp Dijon mustard	4 tbsp vegetable oil
1 tsp fresh rosemary, finely chopped	2 cups fish stock

DIRECTIONS and Cooking Time: 35 Minutes
In a bowl, mix oil, juices, dijon, garlic, salt, and rosemary. Stir well and submerge fish in this mixture. Refrigerate for 1 hour. Meanwhile, heat vegetable oil on Sauté and stir-fry carrot, peas, cherry tomatoes, and okra, for 10 minutes. Add in the fish stock. Seal the lid and cook on Rice for 8 minutes on High. Do a quick release and add in the fish along with half of the marinade. Seal the lid again and cook on Steam for 4 minutes on High. Release the pressure naturally, for 10 minutes. Serve immediately.

Buttery Mackerel With Peppers

INGREDIENTS for Servings: 5

1 tablespoon butter, melted	1/2 teaspoon cayenne pepper
5 mackerel fillets, skin on	1/2 teaspoon dried rosemary
1 green bell pepper, deveined and sliced	Sea salt, to taste
1 red bell pepper, deveined and sliced	1/4 teaspoon ground black pepper, to taste
1 teaspoon marjoram	

DIRECTIONS and Cooking Time: 15 Minutes
Prepare your Electric Pressure Cooker by adding 1 ½ cups of water and steamer basket to its bottom. Season the mackerel fillets with the salt, black pepper, cayenne pepper, rosemary, and marjoram. Place the mackerel fillets in the steamer basket. Drizzle with melted butter. Top with sliced peppers. Secure the lid and choose the "Manual" setting. Cook for 3 minutes at Low pressure. Once cooking is complete, use a quick release; carefully remove the lid. Serve immediately.

Louisiana-style Seafood Boil

INGREDIENTS for Servings: 4

1 cup jasmine rice	1 cup chicken bone broth
1 tablespoon butter	2 bay leaves
1 tablespoon olive oil	1 teaspoon oregano
1/2 pound chicken breasts, cubed	1 teaspoon sage
1 pound shrimp	1 teaspoon basil
2 sweet peppers,	1 teaspoon paprika

deveined and sliced 1 habanero pepper, deveined and sliced 1 onion, chopped 4 cloves garlic, minced	1 tablespoon fish sauce Sea salt and ground black pepper, to taste 1 tablespoon cornstarch

DIRECTIONS and Cooking Time: 25 Minutes
Combine the rice, butter and 1 ½ cups of water in a pot and bring to a rapid boil. Cover and let it simmer on low for 15 minutes. Fluff with a fork and reserve. Press the "Sauté" button and heat the oil. Once hot, cook the chicken breasts for 3 to 4 minutes, stirring periodically. Add the remaining ingredients, except for the cornstarch. Secure the lid. Choose the "Manual" mode and cook for 3 minutes at Low pressure. Once cooking is complete, use a quick pressure release; carefully remove the lid. Mix the cornstarch with 2 tablespoons of cold water. Add the cornstarch slurry to the cooking liquid and stir on the "Sauté" mode until the sauce thickens. Serve over hot jasmine rice. Bon appétit!

Egg Noodles & Cheese With Tuna & Peas

INGREDIENTS for Servings: 4

1 can tuna, drained 3 cups water 4 oz Monterey cheese, grated 16 oz egg noodles ¼ cup breadcrumbs	1 cup frozen peas 28 oz canned mushroom soup Salt and black pepper to taste

DIRECTIONS and Cooking Time: 15 Minutes
Place 3 cups of water and noodles in your IP. Stir in soup, tuna, and frozen peas. Seal the lid, and cook for 5 minutes on Manual at High. When ready, do a quick pressure release. Stir in the cheese. Transfer to a baking dish; sprinkle with breadcrumbs on top. Insert a trivet and 1 cup of water in IP. Put the dish on top, seal lid, and cook 3 minutes on Steam at High. Serve.

Easy Mahi Mahi With Enchilada Sauce

INGREDIENTS for Servings: 2

2 fresh Mahi Mahi fillets ¼ cup commercial enchilada sauce	Salt and pepper, to taste 2 tbsps. butter

DIRECTIONS and Cooking Time: 8 Minutes
Add all the ingredients, except for the butter, to the Electric Pressure Cooker. Lock the lid. Select the Manual mode and cook for 8 minutes at Low Pressure. Once cooking is complete, do a quick pressure release. Carefully open the lid. Stir in the butter and serve on plates.

Beer-steamed Mussels

INGREDIENTS for Servings: 4

3 lb mussels, cleaned and debearded 4 tbsp butter 2 garlic cloves, minced	1 shallots, chopped 2 tbsp parsley, chopped 1 cup beer 1 cup chicken stock

DIRECTIONS and Cooking Time: 15 Minutes
Melt butter in your Electric Pressure Cooker on Sauté. Add in shallots and garlic and cook for 2 minutes. Stir in beer and cook for 1 minute. Mix in stock and mussels and seal the lid. Select Manual and cook for 3 minutes on High pressure. Once ready, perform a quick pressure release and unlock the lid. Discard unopened mussels. Serve sprinkled with parsley.

Lemon & Herbs Stuffed Tench

INGREDIENTS for Servings: 2

1 tench, cleaned and gutted 1 lemon, chopped, quartered 1 tsp fresh rosemary, chopped	2 tbsp olive oil ¼ tsp dried thyme, ground 2 garlic cloves, crushed ½ tsp sea salt

DIRECTIONS and Cooking Time: 20 Minutes
In a bowl, mix olive oil, rosemary, thyme, garlic, and salt. Stir to combine. Brush the fish with the previously prepared mixture and stuff with lemon slices. Pour 4 cups of water into the Electric Pressure Cooker, set the steamer tray and place the fish on top. If the fish is too big and can't fit in, cut in half. Seal the lid and cook on Steam mode for 15 minutes on High Pressure. Do a quick release. For a crispier taste, briefly brown the fish in a grill pan.

Tuna With Egg

INGREDIENTS for Servings: 4

2 cans tuna, drained 2 carrots, peeled and chopped 1 cup frozen peas ¼ cup diced onions 1 can cream of celery soup	2 eggs, beaten ½ cup water ¾ cup milk 2 tbsp butter Salt and ground black pepper to taste

DIRECTIONS and Cooking Time: 25 Minutes
In the Electric Pressure Cooker, combine all of the ingredients and stir to mix. Select the MANUAL setting and set the cooking time for 15 minutes at HIGH pressure. When the timer beeps, use a quick release. Carefully unlock the lid. Serve.

Mussels With Wine-scallion Sauce

INGREDIENTS for Servings: 4

1 ½ pounds frozen mussels, cleaned and debearded 1 cup water 2 tablespoons butter	1 bunch scallion, chopped 1/2 cup cooking wine 2 garlic cloves, sliced

DIRECTIONS and Cooking Time: 10 Minutes
Add the water, wine, and garlic to the inner pot. Add a metal rack to the inner pot. Put the mussels into the steamer basket; lower the steamer basket onto the rack. Secure the lid. Choose the "Steam" mode and cook for 3 minutes at Low pressure. Once cooking is complete, use a quick pressure release; carefully remove the lid. Press the "Sauté" button and add butter and scallions; let it cook until the sauce is thoroughly heated and slightly thickened. Press the "Cancel" button and add the mussels. Serve warm. Bon appétit!

Flounder With Dill And Capers
INGREDIENTS for Servings: 4

1 cup water 1 tbsp. chopped fresh dill 2 tbsps. chopped capers	4 lemon wedges 4 flounder fillets Salt and pepper, to taste

DIRECTIONS and Cooking Time: 10 Minutes
In the Electric Pressure Cooker, set in a steamer basket and pour the water into the pot. Sprinkle salt and pepper to the flounder fillets. Sprinkle with dill and chopped capers on top. Add lemon wedges on top for garnish. Place the fillets on the trivet. Lock the lid. Select the Steam mode and cook for 10 minutes at Low Pressure. Once cooking is complete, do a quick pressure release. Carefully open the lid. Serve warm.

Salmon Zucchini Stew
INGREDIENTS for Servings: 3

½ lb. salmon fillet, cubed ½ tablespoon coconut oil ½ medium onion, chopped ½ garlic clove, minced ½ green bell pepper, seeded and cubed	½ zucchini, sliced ¼ cup tomatoes, chopped ½ cup fish broth 1/8 teaspoon dried oregano, crushed 1/8 teaspoon dried basil, crushed Salt and ground black pepper, to taste

DIRECTIONS and Cooking Time: 6 Hours
Add all the ingredients to the Electric Pressure Cooker and mix well. Secure the lid and select "Slow Cook" for 6 hours. Keep the pressure release handle to the "venting" position. After complete cooking, stir the stew well. Serve immediately.

The Ultimate Crab Patties
INGREDIENTS for Servings: 2

1 cup crab meat ¼ cup black olives, chopped 1 carrot, shredded ½ cup potato mash ¼ cup flour ¼ cup onion, grated 1 ½ cups tomato puree	½ lime, juice and zest 1 tsp cayenne pepper ¼ tsp thyme, dried 1 tbsp olive oil ½ cup chicken broth Salt and black pepper to taste

DIRECTIONS and Cooking Time: 15 Minutes
Place crab meat, carrots, olives, flour, potatoes, lime juice, cayenne pepper, thyme, and onion in a bowl. Mix with hands until fully incorporated. Shape the mixture into two patties. Heat olive oil on Sauté. When hot and sizzling, add the crab cakes and cook for a minute. Flip them over and cook for another minute. Pour tomatoes and broth over and seal lid. Select Manual and set the cooking time to 2 minutes at High. When the timer goes off, do a quick pressure release and serve immediately.

Vermouth Tilapia Medley
INGREDIENTS for Servings: 4

1 pound tilapia fillets, boneless, skinless and diced 2 garlic cloves, minced 1/4 teaspoon freshly ground black pepper, or more to taste 1 cup scallions, chopped 1/2 teaspoon dried oregano 1/2 teaspoon dried basil	1/3 cup dry vermouth 2 cups water 1 teaspoon hot paprika 1 tablespoon fresh lime juice 1 teaspoon dried rosemary 2 tablespoons sesame oil 2 ripe plum tomatoes, crushed Sea salt, to taste 1 cup shellfish stock

DIRECTIONS and Cooking Time: 15 Minutes
Press the "Sauté" button to preheat your Electric Pressure Cooker. Heat the oil and sauté the scallions and garlic until fragrant. Add a splash of vermouth to deglaze the bottom of the inner pot. Secure the lid. Choose the "Manual" mode and High pressure; cook for 5 minutes. Once cooking is complete, use a quick pressure release; carefully remove the lid. Serve with some extra lime slices if desired. Bon appétit!

Greek Kakavia Fish Soup
INGREDIENTS for Servings: 6

12 oz shrimp, deveined 2 cod fillets, skinless, cubed	12 clams 1 tsp thyme, dried 3 bay leaves 1 carrot, chopped

1 can (14.5-oz) tomatoes 2 leeks (white parts only), sliced Salt and black pepper to taste 12 mussels	2 garlic cloves, minced 2 celery stalks, chopped ½ cup dry white wine 4 tbsp lemon juice

DIRECTIONS and Cooking Time: 25 Minutes
Add fish cubes, tomatoes, leeks, shrimp, mussels, clams, thyme, bay leaves, carrot, garlic, celery, white wine, lemon juice, and 6 cups of water to the IP. Stir well. Seal lid, select Manual at High and cook for 5 minutes. When ready, do a quick release. Season with salt and pepper. Remove any unopened clams and mussels; discard bay leaves. Serve in bowls.

Lemon White Fish

INGREDIENTS for Servings: 4

1 tbsp. olive oil 4 white fish fillets Juice and zest of 1 lemon 1 thumb-size ginger, grated	1 cup fish stock Salt and pepper, to taste 4 spring onions, chopped

DIRECTIONS and Cooking Time: 6 Minutes
Except for the spring onions, add all the ingredients to the Electric Pressure Cooker. Lock the lid. Select the Manual mode and set the cooking time for 6 minutes at Low Pressure. Once cooking is complete, do a quick pressure release for 5 minutes. Carefully open the lid. Sprinkle the spring onions on top for garnish before serving.

Mix-and-match Fish Packets

INGREDIENTS for Servings: 4

Sea salt and white pepper, to taste 1/2 pound sugar snap peas, trimmed 2 tablespoons olive oil 2 garlic cloves, minced	1 tablespoon fresh chives, chopped 1 tablespoon fresh parsley, chopped 2 tomatillos, sliced 4 (7-ounces) rainbow trout fillets

DIRECTIONS and Cooking Time: 10 Minutes
Place 1 cup of water and a metal rack in your Electric Pressure Cooker. Place all ingredients in a large sheet of foil. Fold up the sides of the foil to make a bowl-like shape. Lower the fish packet onto the rack. Secure the lid. Choose the "Steam" mode and cook for 3 minutes at Low pressure. Once cooking is complete, use a quick pressure release; carefully remove the lid. Bon appétit!

Tuna With Lemon And Eschalot

INGREDIENTS for Servings: 4

2 eschalots, thinly sliced 1 tablespoon dried parsley flakes 2 tablespoons butter, melted	1 pound tuna fillets 2 lemons, 1 whole and 1 freshly squeezed Sea salt and ground black pepper, to taste

DIRECTIONS and Cooking Time: 10 Minutes
Place 1 cup of water and lemon juice in the Electric Pressure Cooker. Add a steamer basket too. Place the tuna fillets in the steamer basket. Sprinkle the salt, pepper, and parsley over the fish; drizzle with butter and top with thinly sliced eschalots. Secure the lid. Choose the "Steam" mode and Low pressure; cook for 3 minutes. Once cooking is complete, use a quick pressure release; carefully remove the lid. Serve immediately with lemon. Bon appétit!

Herbed Carp Risotto

INGREDIENTS for Servings: 4

Sea salt and ground black pepper, to taste 1 teaspoon dried rosemary, crushed 1/2 teaspoon dried marjoram leaves 1/2 teaspoon dried oregano leaves	1 pound carp, chopped 1 cup chicken stock 1 cup tomato paste 1 cup Arborio rice 1 tablespoon olive oil 1 tablespoon dried parsley

DIRECTIONS and Cooking Time: 15 Minutes
Simply throw all of the above ingredients into your Electric Pressure Cooker. Secure the lid. Choose the "Manual" mode and High pressure; cook for 6 minutes. Once cooking is complete, use a quick pressure release; carefully remove the lid. Serve in individual serving bowls, garnished with fresh lemon slices.

Seafood Paella

INGREDIENTS for Servings: 6

2 cups chopped white fish and scallops 2 cups mussels and shrimp 4 tbsp olive oil 1 onion, diced 1 red bell pepper, diced	1 green bell pepper, diced 2 cups rice A few saffron threads 2 cups fish stock Salt and ground black pepper to taste

DIRECTIONS and Cooking Time: 35 Minutes
Set your Electric Pressure Cooker on SAUTÉ mode, add the oil and heat it up. Add the onion and bell peppers and sauté for 4 minutes. Add the fish, rice, and saffron, stir. Cook for 2 minutes more. Pour in the fish stock and season with salt and pepper, stir. Place the shellfish on top. Press the CANCEL key to stop the SAUTÉ function. Close and lock the lid. Select MANUAL and cook at HIGH pressure for 6 minutes. Once cooking is complete, select CANCEL

and let Naturally Release for 10 minutes. Release any remaining steam manually. Uncover the pot. Stir the dish and let sit for 5 minutes. Serve.

Electric Pressure Cooker Boiled Octopus

INGREDIENTS for Servings: 8

2 ½ pounds whole octopus, sliced and cleaned Salt and pepper to taste	3 tablespoons lemon juice, freshly squeezed 1 cup water

DIRECTIONS and Cooking Time: 15 Minutes
Place all ingredients in the Electric Pressure Cooker. Close the lid and press the Manual button. Adjust the cooking time to 15 minutes. Do quick pressure release.

Delicious Shrimp Salad

INGREDIENTS for Servings: 4

1 pound shrimp, deveined Kosher salt and white pepper, to taste 1 onion, thinly sliced 2 heaping tablespoons fresh parsley, chopped 1 head romaine lettuce, torn into pieces	1 sweet pepper, thinly sliced 1 jalapeno pepper, deseeded and minced 4 tablespoons extra-virgin olive oil 1 lime, juiced and zested 1 tablespoon Dijon mustard

DIRECTIONS and Cooking Time: 15 Minutes
Add a metal trivet and 1 cup of water to your Electric Pressure Cooker. Put the shrimp into the steamer basket. Lower the steamer basket onto the trivet. Secure the lid. Choose the "Steam" mode and cook for 3 minutes at Low pressure. Once cooking is complete, use a quick pressure release; carefully remove the lid. Transfer steamed shrimp to a salad bowl; toss your shrimp with the remaining ingredients and serve well chilled. Bon appétit!

Shrimp Curry

INGREDIENTS for Servings: 2-4

1 lb shrimp, peeled and deveined 2 cups water 8 oz unsweetened coconut milk	1 tbsp garlic, minced 1 tsp curry powder Salt and ground black pepper to taste

DIRECTIONS and Cooking Time: 15 Minutes
Add the water to the Electric Pressure Cooker and insert a steam rack. In a large bowl, combine the shrimp, coconut milk, garlic, and curry powder. Season with salt and pepper. Pour the mixture into the pan and place the dish on the steam rack, uncovered. Close and lock the lid. Select the MANUAL setting and set the cooking time for 4 minutes at LOW pressure. When the timer beeps, use a Quick Release. Carefully unlock the lid. Stir the curry and serve.

Parsley Squid

INGREDIENTS for Servings: 4

2 lb squid, chopped 2 tbsp olive oil Salt and black pepper to taste ½ cup red wine ½ fennel bulb, sliced 1 can (28 oz) crushed tomatoes	1 red onion, sliced 2 garlic cloves, minced 1 tsp Italian seasoning ½ cup parsley, chopped

DIRECTIONS and Cooking Time: 15 Minutes
Mix the olive oil, squid, salt, and pepper in a bowl. Pour the red wine, tomatoes, onion, garlic, rosemary, and fennel in your Electric Pressure Cooker and fit in a steamer basket. Put in the squid and seal the lid. Select Manual and cook for 4 minutes on High pressure. When ready, allow a natural release for 10 minutes, then perform a quick pressure release, and unlock the lid. Serve scattered with parsley.

Shrimp Scampi

INGREDIENTS for Servings: 2-4

1 lb shrimp, peeled and deveined 2 tbsp olive oil 1 clove garlic, minced 1/3 cup tomato paste 10 oz canned tomatoes, chopped 1/3 cup water	¼ tsp oregano, dried 1 tbsp parsley, finely chopped ½ tsp kosher salt ½ tsp ground black pepper to taste 1 cup parmesan, grated

DIRECTIONS and Cooking Time: 15 Minutes
Preheat the Electric Pressure Cooker by selecting SAUTÉ. Add and heat the oil. Add the garlic and sauté for 1 minute. Add the shrimp, tomato paste, tomatoes, water, oregano, parsley, salt and pepper, stir. Close and lock the lid. Select MANUAL and cook at HIGH pressure for 3 minutes. When the timer goes off, use a Quick Release. Carefully open the lid. Sprinkle with parmesan and serve.

Steamed Fish Patra Ni Maachi

INGREDIENTS for Servings: 4

1-pound tilapia fillets	½ cup green commercial chutney

DIRECTIONS and Cooking Time: 10 Minutes
Place a trivet or a steamer basket in the Electric Pressure Cooker. Pour a cup of water. Cut a large parchment paper and place the fish in the middle.3.

Pour over the green chutney. Fold and secure the parchment paper. Place on top of the steamer basket. Close the lid and press the Manual button. Adjust the cooking time to 10 minutes. Do natural pressure release.

Salmon With Green Peas & Rice
INGREDIENTS for Servings: 4

1 cup rice	2 tbsp honey
2 cups vegetable stock	1 tsp sweet paprika
4 skinless salmon fillets	2 jalapeño peppers, seeded and diced
1 cup green peas	4 garlic cloves, minced
3 tbsp olive oil	½ cup canned corn kernels, drained
Salt and black pepper to taste	2 tbsp chopped fresh dill
2 limes, juiced	

DIRECTIONS and Cooking Time: 20 Minutes
Add in rice, stock, and salt. Place a trivet over the rice. In a bowl, mix oil, lime juice, honey, paprika, jalapeño, garlic, and dill. Coat the fish with the honey sauce while reserving a little for garnishing. Lay the salmon fillets on the trivet. Seal the lid and cook on High Pressure for 8 minutes. Do a quick release. Fluff the rice with a fork and mix in the green peas and corn kernels. Transfer to a serving plate and top with the salmon. Drizzle with the remaining honey sauce and enjoy.

Steamed Trout With Garlic & Fresh Herbs
INGREDIENTS for Servings: 2

1 lb fresh trout, (2 pieces)	2 cups fish stock
1 tbsp fresh mint, chopped	3 garlic cloves, chopped
¼ tsp fresh thyme, chopped	3 tbsp olive oil
	2 tbsp fresh lemon juice
1 tbsp fresh parsley, chopped	1 tsp sea salt
	1 tbsp chili

DIRECTIONS and Cooking Time: 30 Minutes
In a bowl, mix mint, thyme, parsley, garlic, olive oil, lemon juice, chili, and salt. Stir to combine. Spread the abdominal cavity of the fish and brush with the marinade. Then, brush the fish from the outside and set aside. Insert the trivet in Electric Pressure Cooker. Pour in the stock and place the trout on top. Seal the lid and cook on Steam mode for 15 minutes on High Pressure. Do a quick release and serve immediately.

Alfredo Tuscan Shrimp
INGREDIENTS for Servings: 3

1 lb. shrimp	1 jar alfredo sauce
1 ½ cups fresh spinach	1 box penne pasta 1 ½ teaspoon Tuscan seasoning
1 cup sun-dried tomatoes	3 cups water

DIRECTIONS and Cooking Time: 15 Minutes
Add the water and pasta to a pot over a medium heat, boil until it cooks completely. Then strain the pasta and keep it aside. Select the "Sauté" function on your Electric Pressure Cooker and add the tomatoes, shrimp, Tuscan seasoning, and alfredo sauce into it. Stir and cook until shrimp turn pink in color. Now add the spinach leaves to the pot and cook for 5 minutes. Add the pasta to the pot and stir well. Serve hot.

Sea Scallops In Champagne Sauce
INGREDIENTS for Servings: 3

1/2 cup champagne	Sea salt and ground black pepper, to taste
2 tablespoons butter	1 pound scallops
1 cup vegetable broth	1/4 teaspoon pink peppercorns, crushed
1/2 teaspoon cayenne pepper	
1 teaspoon ginger garlic paste	

DIRECTIONS and Cooking Time: 10 Minutes
Add all of the above ingredients to the Electric Pressure Cooker. Secure the lid. Choose the "Manual" mode and Low pressure; cook for 3 minutes. Once cooking is complete, use a quick pressure release; carefully remove the lid. Then, press the "Sauté" button and cook the sauce, whisking constantly, until it has reduced by half. Bon appétit!

Soy Sauce Cheese Shrimp Scampi
INGREDIENTS for Servings: 4

2 tbsp butter	Salt and black pepper to taste
1 tbsp Pecorino Romano, grated	For the dipping sauce:
2 shallots, chopped	2 tbsp Soy Sauce
¼ cup white wine	1 tbsp leeks, chopped
1 tsp garlic, minced	½ tbsp olive oil
2 tbsp lemon juice	
1 lb shrimp, deveined	

DIRECTIONS and Cooking Time: 10 Minutes
Melt butter on Sauté in your IP and cook shallots until soft. Add garlic and cook for 1 minute. Stir in wine and cook for another minute. Add the remaining ingredients and stir to combine. Seal lid and cook for 2 minutes on Manual at High. When ready, release the pressure quickly. Serve on a platter with dipping sauce.

Sea Scallops With Champagne Butter Sauce
INGREDIENTS for Servings: 3

1 lb. sea scallops	¼ tsp. pink peppercorns, crushed
1 cup vegetable broth	Sea salt and ground black pepper, to taste
½ cup Champagne	
2 tbsps. butter	
½ tsp. cayenne pepper	

DIRECTIONS and Cooking Time: 5 Minutes
Place all the ingredients in the Electric Pressure Cooker. Lock the lid. Select the Manual mode and set the cooking time for 3 minutes at Low Pressure. Once cooking is complete, do a quick pressure release. Carefully open the lid. Using a slotted spoon, transfer the scallops to a platter and set aside. Set your Electric Pressure Cooker to Sauté and cook the sauce, stirring constantly, or until the sauce is reduced by half. Pour the sauce over the scallops and serve immediately.

Seafood Traditional Spanish Paella
INGREDIENTS for Servings: 4

2 tbsp olive oil	1 tsp turmeric powder
1 onion, chopped	1 pound small clams, scrubbed
4 garlic cloves, minced	1 lb fresh prawns, peeled and deveined
½ cup dry white wine	1 red bell pepper, diced
2 cups rice	1 lemon, cut in wedges
4 cups chicken stock	
1 ½ tsp sweet paprika	
Salt and black pepper to taste	

DIRECTIONS and Cooking Time: 30 Minutes
Stir-fry onion and garlic in a tbsp of oil on Sauté mode for 3 minutes. Pour in wine to deglaze, scraping the bottom of the pot of any brown. Cook for 2 minutes, until the wine is reduced by half. Add in rice and broth. Season with the paprika, turmeric, salt, bell pepper, and pepper. Seal the lid and cook on High Pressure for 10 minutes. Do a quick release. Remove to a plate and wipe the pot clean. Heat the remaining oil on Sauté. Cook clams and prawns for 6 minutes, until the clams have opened and the shrimp are pink. Discard unopened clams. Arrange seafood and lemon wedges over paella, to serve.

Tiger Prawns Paella
INGREDIENTS for Servings: 2-4

1 cup tiger prawns, peeled and deveined	¾ cup risotto rice or paella rice
1 tbsp olive oil	¾ cup green peas, frozen
1 small red onion, roughly chopped	1 cup sweet corn
1 red bell pepper, chopped	1 tbsp fresh parsley, finely chopped
2 chorizo sausage slices	1 tsp salt
2 cups vegetable stock (or chicken stock)	A pinch of saffron threads
	1 whole lemon, quartered

DIRECTIONS and Cooking Time: 30 Minutes
Preheat the Electric Pressure Cooker by selecting SAUTÉ. Add and heat the oil. Add the onion and chorizo slices. Stir and sauté for 3 minute. Add the tiger prawns and cook for 2-3 minutes more, stirring occasionally. Add the rice and stock. Stir well. Add the peas, sweet corn, and parsley. Season with salt and saffron. Close and lock the lid. Select MANUAL and cook at HIGH pressure for 7 minutes. Once pressure cooking is complete, use a Quick Release. Unlock and carefully open the lid. Place the lemon on top. Close the lid and let sit for 10 minutes. Serve.

Sole With Tartar Sauce
INGREDIENTS for Servings: 4

1 tablespoon pickle juice	1/2 cup mayonnaise
2 cloves garlic, smashed	1 teaspoon paprika
1 ½ pounds sole fillets	Sea salt and ground black pepper, to taste

DIRECTIONS and Cooking Time: 10 Minutes
Sprinkle the fillets with salt, black pepper, and paprika. Add 1 ½ cups of water and a steamer basket to the Electric Pressure Cooker. Place the fish in the steamer basket. Secure the lid and choose "Manual" setting. Cook for 3 minutes at Low pressure. Once cooking is complete, use a quick release; carefully remove the lid. Then, make the sauce by mixing the mayonnaise with the pickle juice and garlic. Serve the fish fillets with the well-chilled sauce on the side. Bon appétit!

Vegetable Salmon Skewers
INGREDIENTS for Servings: 4

1 pound salmon, skinned, deboned and cut into bite-sized chunks	1 teaspoon red pepper flakes
1 red onion, cut into wedges	2 tablespoons toasted sesame oil
2 bell peppers, cut into strips	Sea salt and ground black pepper, to taste
8 sticks fresh rosemary, lower leaves removed	1/2 pound yellow squash zucchini, cubed

DIRECTIONS and Cooking Time: 15 Minutes
Prepare your Electric Pressure Cooker by adding 1½ cups of water and metal rack to its bottom. Thread the vegetables and fish alternately onto rosemary sticks. Drizzle with the sesame oil; sprinkle with salt, black pepper, and red pepper flakes. Cover with a piece of foil. Secure the lid. Choose "Manual" mode and Low pressure; cook for 6 minutes. Once cooking is complete, use a quick pressure release; carefully remove the lid. Serve immediately.

Green Lemon Salmon

INGREDIENTS for Servings: 2-4

1 lb salmon fillets, boneless	4 tbsp olive oil
1 lb fresh spinach, torn	2 tbsp lemon juice
2 garlic cloves, chopped	1 tbsp fresh dill, chopped
	1 tsp sea salt
	¼ tsp black pepper

DIRECTIONS and Cooking Time: 30 Minutes
Place spinach in the pot, cover with water and lay the trivet on top. Rub the salmon fillets with half of the olive oil, dill, salt, pepper and garlic. Lay on the trivet. Seal the lid and cook on Steam for 5 minutes on High. Do a quick release. Remove salmon to a serving plate. Drain the spinach in a colander. Serve the fish on a bed of spinach. Season with salt and drizzle with lemon juice.

Spinach & Trout With Red Sauce

INGREDIENTS for Servings: 2

3/4 lb trout fillets	½ tsp fresh rosemary
½ cup fresh spinach, torn	2 tbsp olive oil
2 tomatoes, peeled, diced	¼ cup lime juice
2 cups fish stock	½ tsp sea salt
½ tsp dried thyme	2 garlic cloves, crushed

DIRECTIONS and Cooking Time: 55 Minutes
Rinse the fillets and sprinkle them with sea salt. In a bowl, mix olive oil, thyme, rosemary, and lime juice. Stir well and submerge fillets in this mixture. Refrigerate for 30 minutes; then drain the fillets. Reserve the marinade, grease the pot with 1 tbsp of the marinade and add the fillets and stock. Seal the lid and cook on Steam for 8 minutes on High Pressure. Do a quick release, remove the fish and set aside. Add the remaining marinade to the pot. Hit Sauté and add the tomatoes and spinach. Cook until soft. Give it a good stir and remove to a plate. Add fish, drizzle with tomato sauce and serve warm.

SNACKS & DESSERTS, APPETIZERS RECIPES

Basil Infused Avocado Dip

INGREDIENTS for Servings: 4

2 avocados, sliced	4 tsp lemon juice
¼ cup basil leaves	Salt and black pepper to taste
1 garlic clove, minced	

DIRECTIONS and Cooking Time: 35 Minutes
Place the basil leaves into the cooker, rub the avocado slices with garlic and sprinkle with lemon juice, salt, and pepper. Lay the avocado slices on top of the basil leaves. Add ½ cup of water. Seal the lid, press Manual and cook at High for 15 minutes. After cooking, do a natural pressure release for 10 minutes. Discard the basil and blend the mixture.

Berry Mix, Mango And Apple Sauce

INGREDIENTS for Servings: 2

1 cup mango chunks	1 cup berry mix
2 apples, peeled and diced	¼ cup fresh orange juice
¼ cup almonds, chopped	1 tbsp coconut oil

DIRECTIONS and Cooking Time: 10 Minutes
Pour ½ cup of water, orange juice, and fruits in your IP. Give it a good stir and seal the lid. Press Manual and set the timer to 5 minutes at High. When it goes off, release the pressure quickly. Blend the mixture with a hand blender and immediately stir in the coconut oil. Serve sprinkled with chopped almonds.

Cinnamon-flavored Apple Sauce

INGREDIENTS for Servings: 4

12 apples, chopped	½ tsp nutmeg
1 tsp cinnamon	½ lemon, sliced

DIRECTIONS and Cooking Time: 20 Minutes
Add slices of lemon, ½ cup of water, and apples into the IP. Sprinkle with nutmeg and cinnamon. Seal the lid, select Manual at High, and cook for 3 minutes. When done, release the pressure naturally for 5 minutes. Puree the mixture using an immersion blender. Serve.

Allspices Cake

INGREDIENTS for Servings: 8

1/3 cup almond flour	1 cup pumpkin puree
¾ cup honey	1 tsp almond extract
1 cup raw cashews, chopped	¼ cup coconut oil, melted
1 tsp ground ginger	4 large eggs
½ tsp nutmeg	2 tsp baking powder
1 tsp cinnamon	¼ cup vanilla powder

DIRECTIONS and Cooking Time: 40 Minutes
Grease a baking pan with coconut oil. Mix all the ingredients in a bowl. Gently spread the batter evenly onto the bottom of the baking pan. Add 1 cup of water in the IP and insert a trivet. Put the dish on the trivet. Seal the lid, select Manual at High, and cook for 20 minutes. When done, release the pressure naturally for 5 minutes. Serve sliced.

Easy Peach Cobbler

INGREDIENTS for Servings: 6

6 oz brown sugar	½ tsp nutmeg, freshly grated
3 ½ oz rolled oats	½ tsp allspice, freshly ground
20 oz frozen peach slices	
¼ cup unsalted butter	½ tsp baking powder
¼ tsp kosher salt	4 oz flour

DIRECTIONS and Cooking Time: 35 Minutes
Combine baking powder, sugar, oats, flour, nutmeg, allspice, and salt in a bowl. Add the butter and beat it into the ingredients until there is a crumbly texture. Fold in the peach slices. Grease the bottom as well as the sides of a baking dis with butter. Add in the mixture. Pour 1 cup of water into the IP and fit in a trivet. Place the baking dish on top. Seal the lid and press Manual. Cook at High for 15 minutes. After cooking, do a quick pressure release. Let it cool and serve.

Cheesy Breakfast Potatoes

INGREDIENTS for Servings: 8

3 russet potatoes, diced	1 (10.75-oz) can chicken soup
1 green bell pepper, diced	¼ tsp basil, dried
	¼ tsp oregano, dried
1 red bell pepper, diced	½ cup sour cream
	1 ½ cups cheddar, shredded
2 tbsp parsley, chopped	1 onion, diced
Salt and black pepper to taste	1 lb smoked chicken sausages, sliced

DIRECTIONS and Cooking Time: 35 Minutes
Combine potatoes, sausage, bell peppers, sour cream, onion, basil, oregano, and cheese in the IP. Pour in chicken soup along with salt and pepper. Seal lid, select Manual at High, and cook for 8 minutes. Do a quick release. Serve hot, garnished with parsley.

Duck Legs With Serrano Pepper Sauce

INGREDIENTS for Servings: 6

1 ½ lb duck legs ½ cup maple syrup ½ cup tomato puree 2 tsp basil 1 tbsp oregano 1 tbsp cumin Salt and black pepper to taste	Sauce: ½ cup whipping cream ½ cup chopped parsley ¼ cup olive oil 2 tbsp lemon juice 2 serrano peppers, chopped 1 garlic clove

DIRECTIONS and Cooking Time: 40 Minutes
Pour 1 ½ cups of water in the pressure cooker and place duck legs in a baking pan. In a bowl, combine all the remaining duck ingredients and pour over the meat. Put the baking pan on top of inserted rack. Seal the lid. Cook on Manual for 20 minutes at High. Release pressure naturally for 10 minutes. Pulse all sauce ingredients in a food processor and transfer to a Servings bowl. Serve duck bites with the sauce.

Cauliflower Popcorn
INGREDIENTS for Servings: 6

10 oz cauliflower, florets 1 tbsp olive oil	Salt and black pepper to taste

DIRECTIONS and Cooking Time: 15 Minutes
In a bowl, sprinkle florets with salt and olive oil. Add 1 cup of water into the IP. Place trivet inside. Put florets in a baking pan and place on top of the trivet. Seal the lid and press Manual. Cook for 5 minutes at High. After cooking, do a quick pressure release. Serve.

Spinach Dip
INGREDIENTS for Servings: 4

2 cups spinach, chopped 1 garlic clove, minced 1/3 cup coconut milk	1 oz cooked bacon, chopped 1/3 white onion, chopped

DIRECTIONS and Cooking Time: 15 Minutes
Add spinach, garlic, onion, bacon, and coconut milk to the IP. Pour in ½ cup of water. Seal the lid and press Manual. Cook at High for 4 minutes. After cooking, do a quick pressure release. Transfer to a Servings dishes.

Peanut Pear Wedges
INGREDIENTS for Servings: 3

2 pears, cut into wedges	3 tbsp peanut butter 2 tbsp olive oil

DIRECTIONS and Cooking Time: 5 Minutes
Pour 1 cup of water in the pressure cooker. Place the pear wedges in a steamer basket and then lower the basket at the bottom. Seal the lid, and cook for 2 minutes on Manual at High. When the timer goes off, do a quick pressure release. Remove the basket, discard the water, and wipe the cooker clean. Press the Sauté and heat the oil. Add the pear wedges and cook until browned. Top with peanut butter to serve.

Coconut & Orange Cheesecake
INGREDIENTS for Servings: 4

For the crust: 1 ¾ cups crumbled crackers ½ cup butter, melted ¼ cup coconut sugar A pinch salt For the filling: 2 eggs 8 oz heavy cream	½ cup coconut sugar 1 ¾ cups cold milk 2 tbsp orange zest ¼ cup orange juice 3 tbsp cornstarch 2 cups of water Topping: 3 oranges, sliced thinly

DIRECTIONS and Cooking Time: 45 Minutes
Line the bottom of a cake pan with aluminum foil, then grease with cooking spray. In a bowl, mix the crust ingredients. Spoon the crust into the cake pan and press firmly into the bottom. Chill for 20 minutes in the freezer. In a bowl, beat eggs with heavy cream and sugar. Whisk in milk, orange zest, orange juice, and cornstarch until smooth. Remove the crust from the fridge and pour the filling over. Pour 1 cup of water in your IP and insert a trivet. Place the cake pan on top. Seal the lid, select Manual at High for 35 minutes. When ready, naturally release the pressure for 10 minutes, then a quick pressure release, and open the lid. Carefully remove the cake pan and let cool at room temperature. Once cooled, refrigerate for 8 hours or more. Before Servings, top with the blood orange slices, and slice into wedges. Serve.

Beef Ribs Texas Bbq Style
INGREDIENTS for Servings: 4

1 cup BBQ sauce 2 tbsp Ancho chili powder ½ tbsp garlic powder 2 tbsp olive oil	½ yellow onion, diced 2 lb beef ribs, cut into 2-bone pieces Salt and black pepper to taste

DIRECTIONS and Cooking Time: 1 Hour
Set your IP to Sauté and heat the olive oil. Rub the beef with salt, pepper, garlic, and chili powder and brown on all the sides for 5-6 minutes. Set aside. To the pot, add the onion and cook for 3 minutes. Return the beef, pour in the BBQ sauce, and a ½ cup of water. Seal lid, select Manual at High, and cook for 45 minutes. When ready, release the pressure naturally for 10 minutes. Serve hot.

Lemony Berry Cream
INGREDIENTS for Servings: 2

½ cup blueberries ½ cup strawberries, chopped ½ cup raspberries	1 cup milk ¼ tsp vanilla extract ¼ tsp lemon zest

DIRECTIONS and Cooking Time: 4 Hours And 5 Minutes
Place all ingredients, except for the vanilla extract, inside your pressure cooker. Seal the lid, select Steam, and set the timer to 3 minutes at High. When it goes off, do a quick pressure release. Remove to a blender. Add vanilla extract and pulse until smooth. Divide between two Servings glasses and cool for 4 hours before Servings .

Simple Cranberry Chocolate Biscuits
INGREDIENTS for Servings: 4

4 peaches, halved lengthwise 8 dried cranberries, chopped 4 tbsp pecans, chopped	1 cup crumbled cookies 1 tsp cinnamon powder ¼ tsp grated nutmeg ¼ tsp ground cloves

DIRECTIONS and Cooking Time: 20 Minutes
Pour 2 cups of water into the pressure cooker and add a trivet. Arrange the peaches on a greased baking dish cut-side-up. To prepare the filling, mix all of the remaining ingredients. Stuff the peaches with the mixture. Cover with aluminium foil and lower it onto the trivet. Seal the lid, press Manual, and cook for 15 minutes at High. Do a quick pressure release.

Swiss Chard Crisps With Orange Juice
INGREDIENTS for Servings: 4

Salt and black pepper to taste 3 garlic cloves, minced	1 lb Swiss chard 1 tbsp olive oil 2 tbsp orange juice

DIRECTIONS and Cooking Time: 15 Minutes
Wash Swiss chard and remove the stems. Set your IP to Sauté and heat oil. Cook garlic for a minute, or until fragrant. Add in the Swiss chard and ½ cup of water. Seal the lid. Cook on Manual for 6 minutes at High. Do a quick release, and drizzle with orange juice.

Herby Cipollini Onions
INGREDIENTS for Servings: 6

1 ½ lb cippolini onions, peeled 2 tbsp lemon juice 3 tbsp olive oil ½ tsp rosemary, chopped	2 bay leaves 1 tsp lemon zest 2 tbsp fresh parsley Salt and black pepper to taste

DIRECTIONS and Cooking Time: 15 Minutes
Combine 1 cup of water, onions, and bay leaves in your IP. Seal the lid, press Manual, and cook for 6 minutes at High. Do a quick release. Drain the onions and transfer them a cutting board. Cut into quarters. Whisk together the remaining ingredients and pour over the onions.

Pineapple Chocolate Pudding
INGREDIENTS for Servings: 4

1 lime, zested, grated ½ cup pineapple juice 2 oz chocolate, chopped ¼ cup sugar 2 tbsp butter, softened	¼ cup cornstarch 1 cup almond milk A pinch of salt ½ tsp ginger, caramelized 3 eggs, yolks & whites separated

DIRECTIONS and Cooking Time: 30 Minutes
Combine sugar, cornstarch, salt, and butter in a bowl. Mix in pineapple juice and grated lime zest. Add in the egg yolks, ginger, almond milk, and whisk to mix well. Stir in egg whites. Pour this mixture into custard cups and cover with aluminium foil. Add 1 ½ cups of water to the pressure cooker. Place a trivet into the pressure cooker, and lower the cups onto the rack. Select Manual and cook for 25 minutes at High. Once the cooking is over, do a quick pressure release. Carefully open the lid and stir in the chocolate. Serve chilled.

Holiday Almond Cake
INGREDIENTS for Servings: 4

3 eggs, yolks & whites separated ¾ cup almond flour 1 ½ cups warm coconut milk	½ tsp almond extract ½ cup almond sugar 2 tbsp coconut oil, melted

DIRECTIONS and Cooking Time: 50 Minutes
In a bowl, beat in the egg yolks along with the almond sugar. In a separate bowl, beat the whites until soft form peaks. Stir in almond extract and coconut oil. Gently fold in the almond flour. Line a baking dish and pour the batter inside. Cover with aluminum foil. Pour 1 cup of water in your pressure cooker and add a wire rack. Lower the dish onto the rack. Seal the lid, select Manual, and cook for 40 minutes at High. Do a quick pressure release, and serve.

Thyme Tomato Sauce
INGREDIENTS for Servings: 16

3 lb tomatoes, peeled and diced 1 cup green onions, chopped ¼ cup olive oil	½ tsp dried basil ½ tsp dried oregano 2 cloves garlic, minced ½ tsp dried thyme

| 2 tsp brown sugar | Salt and black pepper |
| 1 green chili, chopped | to taste |

DIRECTIONS and Cooking Time: 25 Minutes
Select Sauté on your IP and heat the oil; cook the green onions and garlic until tender, for about 3 minutes. Add the remaining ingredients and ½ cup of water. Seal the lid, select Manual, and cook for 10 minutes at High. Do a quick pressure release. Let cool before Servings.

Almond Butter Lemon Pears

INGREDIENTS for Servings: 2

| 2 pears, cut into wedges | ½ tsp cinnamon |
| ½ cup lemon juice | 1 tbsp almond butter |

DIRECTIONS and Cooking Time: 10 Minutes
Combine lemon juice and 1 cup of water in the pressure cooker. Place the pear wedges in the steamer basket and lower the basket into the cooker. Seal the lid, select Manual, and cook for 3 minutes at High. Release the pressure quickly. Open the lid and remove the steamer basket. Transfer the pear wedges to a bowl. Drizzle with almond butter and sprinkle with cinnamon.

Apple Coconut Dessert

INGREDIENTS for Servings: 2

| ¼ cup flour | 1 cup coconut milk |
| 2 apples, peeled and diced | ¼ cup shredded coconut |

DIRECTIONS and Cooking Time: 10 Minutes
Combine all ingredients in the pressure cooker. Seal the lid, select Manual, and set the timer to 5 minutes at High. When ready, do a quick pressure release. Divide the mixture between two bowls.

Tasty Apple Risotto

INGREDIENTS for Servings: 8

¼ cup butter	1/8 tsp nutmeg
1/3 cup brown sugar	1 ½ tsp cinnamon
1 ½ cups rice	3 apples, peeled and diced
Salt and black pepper to taste	4 cups milk

DIRECTIONS and Cooking Time: 50 Minutes
Turn the IP on Sauté and melt the butter. Add in the rice and stir, making sure to coat it evenly. Add the apples, sugar, and spices, and stir in the milk. Seal the lid, select Manual at High, and cook for 20 minutes. When ready, perform natural pressure release for 15 minutes, then quick pressure release.

Awesome Chocolate Lava Cake

INGREDIENTS for Servings: 4

2 tbsp butter, melted	1 tsp vanilla extract
1 cup chocolate, melted	3 eggs plus 1 yolk, beaten
6 tbsp coconut flour	¾ cup coconut sugar

DIRECTIONS and Cooking Time: 15 Minutes
Combine all ingredients in a bowl. Grease 4 ramekins with cooking spray. Divide the filling between the ramekins. Pour 1 cup of water in your IP and put a trivet. Place the ramekins on the trivet. Seal the lid and cook for 10 minutes Manual at High. When ready, do a quick pressure release. Serve.

Rose Rice Pudding With Nuts

INGREDIENTS for Servings: 4

1 cup basmati rice	¼ cup raisins
1 ½ cups milk	Pumpkin seeds for topping
1 cup water	
½ cup sugar	¼ cup chopped pecans and cashews
½ tsp rose essence	
A pinch salt	

DIRECTIONS and Cooking Time: 25 Minutes
In your IP, put the rice, milk, water, sugar, rose essence, salt, raisins, pecans and cashews, and stir. Seal the lid, select Manual, and cook for 20 minutes at High. Perform a natural pressure release, for about 5 minutes. Stir the pudding and serve garnished with pumpkin seeds.

Sausage & Cream Cheese Dip

INGREDIENTS for Servings: 6

| 1 lb bulk sausages | 8 oz cream cheese |
| 1 can (14.5-oz) tomatoes with chilies | 2 tbsp olive oil |

DIRECTIONS and Cooking Time: 38 Minutes
Heat olive oil on Sauté and brown the sausages for 6-8 minutes. Stir in the tomatoes and cream cheese. Add in 1 cup of water. Seal the lid and press Manual. Cook for 25 minutes at High. After cooking, do a quick pressure release. Serve dip with crackers.

Teriyaki Chicken In Lettuce Wrap

INGREDIENTS for Servings: 6

3 garlic cloves, minced	½ tbsp ground ginger
4 chicken breasts, cubed	½ cup coconut milk
	½ cup honey
¼ tbsp red wine vinegar	1 onion, chopped
	1 ¼ cups water
1 tbsp arrowroot powder	6 lettuce leaves
	Shredded cheddar cheese for garnish

DIRECTIONS and Cooking Time: 36 Minutes
Except for the lettuce leaves, cheese and arrowroot powder, mix the other ingredients in your IP. Seal the

lid, select Manual at High, and cook for 18 minutes. When ready, release the pressure naturally for 5 minutes. In a bowl, mix water and arrowroot powder. Remove the chicken from cooker and set aside. Add the arrowroot slurry to the cooker and cook for 3 minutes on Sauté. Add the chicken back to cooker and stir. Serve on lettuce leaves topped with cheese.

Yummy Smoked Sausages

INGREDIENTS for Servings: 4

| 1 lb smoked sausage, sliced | 1 onion, diced |
| ½ cup brown sugar | ½ cup ketchup |

DIRECTIONS and Cooking Time: 25 Minutes
Place all the ingredients in the IP. Stir to coat sausages. Pour in 1 cup of water. Seal the lid and press Manual. Cook at High for 20 minutes. After cooking, do a quick pressure release. Serve sausage on toothpicks as a tasty appetizer.

Party Cinnamon & Yogurt Cheesecake

INGREDIENTS for Servings: 8

2 eggs	1 tsp cinnamon
¼ cup sugar	1 ½ cups graham cracker crumbs
1 ½ cups yogurt	
4 oz cream cheese, softened	4 tbsp butter, melted

DIRECTIONS and Cooking Time: 40 Minutes
Mix the butter and cracker crumbs, and press the mixture onto the bottom of a springform pan. In a bowl, beat cream cheese with yogurt, cinnamon, and sugar. Beat in the eggs one at a time. Spread the filling on top of the crust. Pour 1 cup of water in your cooker and add a trivet. Lower the pan onto the trivet. Lock the lid, press Manual for 35 minutes at High. Once cooking is completed, do a quick pressure release. Let cool and refrigerate for 6 hours.

Christmas Banana Bread

INGREDIENTS for Servings: 12

3 ripe bananas, mashed	1 tbsp pineapple juice
1 ¼ cups sugar	1 stick butter, softened
1 cup milk	A pinch of salt
2 cups all-purpose flour	¼ tsp cinnamon
1 tsp baking soda	½ tsp pure vanilla extract
1 tsp baking powder	

DIRECTIONS and Cooking Time: 45 Minutes
In a bowl, mix together flour, baking powder, baking soda, sugar, vanilla, and salt. Add in bananas, cinnamon, and pineapple juice. Slowly stir in the butter and milk. Give it a good stir until everything is well combined. Pour the batter into a medium-sized round pan. Place a trivet at the bottom of the pressure cooker and fill with 2 cups of water. Place the pan on the trivet. Select Manual and cook for 40 minutes at High. Do a quick pressure release. Let cool before slicing.

Dijon Deviled Eggs

INGREDIENTS for Servings: 4

4 eggs	Salt and black pepper to taste
1 tsp chili pepper	
1 tbsp mayonnaise	Fresh parsley, for garnish
1 tsp Dijon mustard	
1 tbsp pickle juice	

DIRECTIONS and Cooking Time: 20 Minutes
Place the eggs and 1 cup of water in your pressure cooker. Seal the lid and cook on Manual for 5 minutes at High. Once cooking is over, do a quick pressure release. Place the eggs in an ice bath and let cool for 5 minutes. Peel and cut them in half. Remove yolks to a mixing dish and mash with a fork; add the remaining ingredients, excluding the parsley and stir. Fill the egg halves with the yolk mixture. Sprinkle with parsley.

Best Bacon Wrapped Mini Smokies

INGREDIENTS for Servings: 12

| 1 lb bacon slices | 2 tbsp vinegar |
| 14 oz mini smokie sausages | ¾ cup brown sugar |

DIRECTIONS and Cooking Time: 35 Minutes
Cut the bacon slices in half. Wrap a slice of bacon around each individual sausage. Put the seam side facing down in a baking dish. In a small bowl, mix vinegar and brown sugar. Drizzle this mixture over smokies in the dish. Place in the fridge overnight. Pour 1 cup of water into the IP and fit in a trivet. Remove the smokies from fridge and place the dish on the trivet. Seal the lid and press Manual. Cook at High for 20 minutes. After cooking, do a quick release.

Cheesy Hamburger Dip

INGREDIENTS for Servings: 6

3 ½ lb ground beef	6 tortilla chips
1 onion, finely chopped	1 jar (16-oz) chunky pace salsa
1 box Velveeta cheese, cubed	3 tbsp olive oil

DIRECTIONS and Cooking Time: 40 Minutes
Heat olive oil on Sauté and brown the meat for 8-10 minutes. Add onions at the 5th minutes of the meat cooking and mix well. Add salsa, 1 cup of water, and cheese cubes and stir. Seal the lid and press Poultry. Cook for 20 minutes at High. After cooking, do a quick pressure release. Serve with tortilla chips.

Almond Butter Bars

INGREDIENTS for Servings: 6

1 cup flour	1 cup oats
1 egg	½ cup sugar
½ cup almond butter, softened	½ tsp baking soda
	½ tsp salt
½ cup butter, softened	½ cup brown sugar

DIRECTIONS and Cooking Time: 55 Minutes
Beat the eggs, almond butter, butter, salt, white sugar, and brown sugar. Fold in the oats, flour, and baking soda. Press the batter into a greased baking pan. Cover with a piece of foil. Pour 1 cup of water into the IP and add a trivet. Lower the pan onto the trivet. Seal the lid. Press Manual and cook for 35 minutes at High. When ready, do a quick release. Cool for 15 minutes, invert onto a plate, and cut into bars.

Mayonnaise & Bacon Stuffed Eggs

INGREDIENTS for Servings: 4

2 oz fried bacon, chopped	8 eggs
	1 tsp mayonnaise
Salt and black pepper to taste	Chopped chives for garnish

DIRECTIONS and Cooking Time: 23 Minutes
Place eggs into the IP and cover with water. Seal the lid and press Manual. Cook at High for 8 minutes. After cooking, do a quick pressure release. Remove eggs and carefully put them in a bowl of ice water for 5 minutes. Peel off the eggshells. Cut eggs in half and remove the yolks. In a bowl, mix egg yolks, mayo, salt, pepper, and fried bacon. Stir to combine well. Fill the egg white with egg yolk mixture, top with chives for garnish.

Pineapple Upside Down Cake

INGREDIENTS for Servings: 6

1 cup flour	½ cup heavy cream
½ cup pecans, chopped	2 tbsp whole milk
	1 tsp pure vanilla extract
½ tsp ground cinnamon	
¾ tsp baking powder	2 large eggs
½ cup light brown sugar	2 tbsp dark rum
	½ ripe pineapple, sliced
10 tbsp butter, softened	1 tbsp chopped maraschino cherries
¼ tsp grated nutmeg	Some whole maraschino cherries for garnish
¼ tsp fine salt	
2/3 cup sugar	
1 tbsp confectioners' sugar	

DIRECTIONS and Cooking Time: 70 Minutes
Grease a baking dish with cooking spray. Line it with a double layer of foil, then grease the foil. Add in brown sugar and rum. Arrange the pineapple slices on the bottom of the baking dish, pressing into the sugar mixture. In a bowl, mix flour, pecans, baking powder, cinnamon, nutmeg, and salt. In another bowl, combine sugar and butter, and using a mixer, beat until fluffy. Scrape down sides of a bowl with butter mixture, then whisk in the eggs and vanilla. Add in the milk and continue beating until smooth. Spread the batter over the pineapples. Pour 1 cup of water in the IP and insert a trivet. Put the dish on the trivet. Seal the lid, select Manual at High, and cook for 30 minutes. When done, perform a natural pressure release for 10 minutes, then a quick pressure release to let out the remaining steam. Allow the cake to rest for 20 minutes. Carefully, invert cake onto a platter and peel off the foil. Whip the cream until peaks form. Fold in the confectioners' sugar and chopped cherries. Serve cake slices with a nice dollop of whipped cream and a whole cherry on top.

Amazing White Chocolate Fondue

INGREDIENTS for Servings: 12

10 oz white chocolate, chopped	8 oz cream cheese
	¼ tsp cinnamon powder
2 tsp coconut liqueur	A pinch of salt

DIRECTIONS and Cooking Time: 10 Minutes
Melt the chocolate in a heatproof recipient. Add the remaining ingredients, except for the liqueur. Transfer this recipient to the metal trivet. Pour 1 cup of water into the cooker, and fit in the trivet. Seal the lid, select Manual, and cook for 5 minutes at High. Do a quick pressure release. Pull out the container with tongs. Mix in the coconut liqueur and serve with fresh fruits.

Cashew Cholocate Spread

INGREDIENTS for Servings: 16

1 ¼ lb cashews, halved	1 tsp vanilla extract
	¼ tsp cardamom, grated
½ cup cocoa powder	
½ cups icing sugar, sifted	¼ tsp cinnamon powder
	½ tsp grated nutmeg

DIRECTIONS and Cooking Time: 30 Minutes
Put cashews in a blender and blitz until you obtain a paste. Place in the cooker along with the remaining ingredients and 10 oz of water. Seal the lid, select Manual, and cook for 13 minutes at High. Once ready, allow for a natural pressure release for 10 minutes.

Apricot, Pear And Cherry Compote

INGREDIENTS for Servings: 5

1 ½ cups apricots, dried	1 tsp orange zest
	½ cup white wine

4 ripe pears, chopped	1 1/3 cups sugar
Pinch of salt	2 ¼ cups hot water
¼ tsp vanilla extract	1 cup cherries, dried

DIRECTIONS and Cooking Time: 20 Minutes
Mix sugar, water, zest, vanilla, wine, and salt in your IP until the sugar is dissolved. Gently stir in the fruits, and make sure not to squish the pears. Seal the lid, select Manual at High, and cook for 10 minutes. Do a quick release. Allow to cool and serve.

Apple Coffee Cake

INGREDIENTS for Servings: 4

2 cups baking mix	2 tbsp butter, melted
2/3 cup applesauce	2 tbsp sugar
¼ cup milk	Topping:
1 egg	¼ cup baking mix
1 tsp vanilla extract	¼ cup nuts, chopped
1 tsp ground cinnamon	2 tbsp butter, softened
2 apples, peeled and diced	¼ cup brown sugar

DIRECTIONS and Cooking Time: 37 Minutes
Grease a baking dish with cooking spray. Combine the applesauce, milk, baking mix, sugar, butter, apples, vanilla, cinnamon, and egg in a bowl. Mix the batter until thick and lumpy. In another bowl, combine the topping ingredients. Pour the batter into the baking dish and spread the topping evenly. Pour 1 cup of water in your IP and insert a trivet. Place the dish on top. Seal the lid, select Manual at High, and cook for 12 minutes. Do a quick release. Let cool for a few minutes before Servings .

Cheese Sweet Corn

INGREDIENTS for Servings: 6

Juice of 2 limes	6 tbsp yogurt
1 cup Grana Padano, grated	½ tsp garlic powder
6 ears sweet corn	Salt and black pepper to taste

DIRECTIONS and Cooking Time: 10 Minutes
Pour in 1 cup of water and add a trivet. Put the corn on top. Seal the lid, and cook on Steam for 3 minutes at High. Combine the remaining ingredients, except for the cheese in a bowl. Once done, do a quick pressure release. Let cool for a couple of minutes. Remove husks from the corn and brush them with the mixture. Sprinkle Grana Padano cheese on top and serve.

Fall Root Vegetable Mix

INGREDIENTS for Servings: 4

1 ½ lb mixed root vegetables	1 cup vegetable broth
	2 tbsp olive oil
	A pinch of salt

3 garlic cloves, minced	2 tbsp parsley, chopped
1 onion, sliced	

DIRECTIONS and Cooking Time: 25 Minutes
Heat olive oil on Sauté in the IP and cook onion and garlic for 3 minutes. Cut all the root vegetables into small pieces, and add them to the cooker along with salt and broth. Seal the lid, press Manual, and cook for 7 minutes at High. After cooking, do a quick pressure release. Serve hot sprinkled with parsley.

Chocolate Pudding Cake

INGREDIENTS for Servings: 8

3 cups milk	1 cup fresh strawberries
1 cup whipped cream	
1 box (19-oz) chocolate fudge cake mix	1 (14-oz) package chocolate instant pudding

DIRECTIONS and Cooking Time: 35 Minutes
In a bowl, mix together milk and pudding mix until smooth. Add the mixture to a greased baking dish. Prepare the cake batter according to the box directions. Pour it over the pudding, do not stir. Add 1 cup of water in the IP and insert a trivet. Put the dish on the trivet. Seal the lid, select Manual at High, and cook for 25 minutes. When done, do a quick release. Let cool. Top with whipped cream and strawberries and slice.

Smoked Paprika Potato Chips

INGREDIENTS for Servings: 4

4 russet potatoes, sliced	Salt and black pepper to taste
½ tsp smoked paprika	2 tbsp olive oil

DIRECTIONS and Cooking Time: 20 Minutes
Place the slices in the pressure cooker and pour enough water to cover them. Seal the lid, select Manual, and set the timer to 10 minutes at High. Release the pressure quickly. Drain the potatoes and discard the water. Transfer to a bowl. Wipe the cooker clean. Press Sauté, set to High, and heat the oil. Sprinkle the potatoes with paprika, salt, and pepper, and toss to combine. Be careful not to break them. When the oil is hot, add the potatoes and cook for about a minute, per side.

Pumpkin Hummus

INGREDIENTS for Servings: 5

2 lb pumpkin, chopped	½ tsp garlic, minced
	3 tbsp olive oil
1 tbsp pumpkin seeds	1 tsp tahini sauce
1/3 tsp salt	
½ tsp cayenne pepper	

DIRECTIONS and Cooking Time: 25 Minutes

Pour 1 cup of water into the IP and insert a trivet inside. Place the pumpkin in a pan on top of the trivet. Seal the lid and press Manual. Cook at High for 15 minutes. After cooking, do a quick pressure release. Let the pumpkin cool, then transfer to a blender and add olive oil and tahini. Add garlic, cayenne pepper, salt and pumpkin seeds. Blend the mixture for a few minutes, or until smooth. Transfer to bowls and serve.

Quick Rum Egg Custard

INGREDIENTS for Servings: 4

1 egg + 2 egg yolks	½ tsp pure rum extract
½ cup sugar	½ tsp vanilla extract
½ cups milk	
2 cups heavy cream	

DIRECTIONS and Cooking Time: 15 Minutes
Beat egg and egg yolks in a bowl. Gently add pure rum extract and vanilla extract. Mix in milk and heavy cream. Stir and add the sugar. Pour this mixture into 4 ramekins. Add 1 cup of water, insert a trivet, and lay the ramekins on the trivet. Select Manual and cook for 10 minutes at High. Do a quick pressure release.

Silky Lemon Cheesecake With Blueberries

INGREDIENTS for Servings: 6

1 ½ cups graham cracker crust	½ stick butter, melted
1 cup blueberries	¾ cup sugar
3 cups cream cheese	1 tsp vanilla paste
1 tbsp fresh lemon juice	1 tsp finely grated lemon zest
3 eggs	

DIRECTIONS and Cooking Time: 25 Minutes
Insert a trivet into the pressure cooker and add 1 ½ cups of water. Grease a springform. Mix in graham cracker crust with sugar and butter in a bowl. Press the mixture to form a crust at the bottom. Blend the blueberries and cream cheese with an electric mixer. Crack in the eggs and keep mixing until well combined. Mix in the remaining ingredients, and give it a good stir. Pour this mixture into the pan, and cover the pan with aluminium foil. Lay the springform pan on the trivet. Select Manual and cook for 20 minutes at High. Once the cooking is complete, do a quick pressure release. Refrigerate the cheesecake for at least 2 hours.

Zesty Carrots With Pistachios

INGREDIENTS for Servings: 4

2 lb carrots, cut into rounds	¼ cup raisins
½ cup pistachios, chopped	Salt and black pepper to taste
1 tbsp butter	1 tbsp vinegar

DIRECTIONS and Cooking Time: 15 Minutes
Select Sauté and melt the butter. Add in carrots and cook for 5 minutes until tender. Add raisins, 1 cup of water, and salt. Seal the lid, press Manual, and cook for 3 minutes at High. When done, do a quick pressure release. Pour in vinegar, and black pepper, and give it a good stir. Scatter the pistachios over the top and serve.

Mom's Banana Cake

INGREDIENTS for Servings: 6

Banana:	½ tsp ground cinnamon
6 tbsp butter, cubed	¼ tsp ground nutmeg
6 bananas, halved lengthwise	2 tbsp whole milk
3 tbsp dark rum	1 egg yolk
¾ cup dark brown sugar	2/3 cups sugar
Cake:	4 tbsp butter, softened
¾ tsp baking soda	¼ tsp fine salt
¾ cups cake flour	Ice cream for Servings

DIRECTIONS and Cooking Time: 1 Hour And 25 Minutes
Grease a baking pan with cooking spray and line with foil. Sprinkle some butter, rum, and brown sugar on top. Cover with banana halves, with cut side down. Sift flour, baking powder, cinnamon, nutmeg, and salt into a large bowl; then whisk to combine. In another bowl, beat butter and sugar with electric mixer until light and fluffy. Add the egg yolk to butter mixture and beat until well blended. Fold in flour mixture. Add the milk in 2 parts and mix at medium speed to make a smooth batter. Pour batter over bananas and smooth with a spatula. Pour 1 cup of water in the IP and insert a trivet. Put the dish on the trivet. Seal the lid, select Manual at High, and cook for 30 minutes. When done, release the pressure naturally for 5 minutes. Let cool. Lift the cake onto a platter using the foil. Remove the foil and carefully invert the cake onto a Servings platter. Serve with ice cream.

Chocolate-strawberry Bars

INGREDIENTS for Servings: 6

| ½ cup almond butter | 2 tbsp cocoa powder |
| 2 cups strawberries | |

DIRECTIONS and Cooking Time: 20 Minutes
Place strawberries and almond butter in a bowl and mash with a fork. Add in cocoa powder and stir until well combined. Pour the strawberry and almond butter in a greased baking dish. Pour 1 cup of water in the pressure cooker and lower a trivet. Place the baking dish on top of the trivet and seal the lid. Select Manual and cook for 15 minutes at High. When it goes off, do a quick release. Let cool before cutting into squares.

Sticky Sweet Chicken Wings

INGREDIENTS for Servings: 5

2 pounds chicken wings	1/3 cup balsamic vinegar
Salt and black pepper to taste	1/3 cup soy sauce
3 garlic cloves, minced	1 ½ tsp Sriracha sauce
1 tbsp fresh lime juice	1 tsp ground coriander
¼ cup chicken broth	3 tbsp potato starch
1/3 cup raw honey	¼ cup fresh cilantro for garnish

DIRECTIONS and Cooking Time: 38 Minutes
Season the chicken wings with salt and pepper, and place in your IP. In a bowl, combine honey, broth, vinegar, soy sauce, garlic, lime juice, coriander and sriracha sauce and mix well. Pour mixture over the chicken wings and toss to coat. Seal the lid, select Manual at High, and cook for 20 minutes. Perform a natural pressure release for 5 minutes. Whisk potato starch with ¼ cup of cold water until smooth, then stir in the pot. Cook for an additional 2-3 minutes on Sauté. Serve hot with chopped cilantro leaves.

Bacon Asparagus Wraps

INGREDIENTS for Servings: 4

1 lb asparagus, trimmed	Salt and black pepper to taste
3 oz bacon slices	

DIRECTIONS and Cooking Time: 14 Minutes
Pour 1 cup of water in the IP and insert a trivet. Season the asparagus with salt and pepper, then wrap in bacon slices. Place wraps on the trivet and lock the lid. Press Manual and cook for 4 minutes at High. After cooking, do a quick pressure release to release all the steam and unlock lid. Serve warm.

Tasty Honey Pumpkin Pie

INGREDIENTS for Servings: 4

1 lb pumpkin, diced	½ tsp cinnamon
1 egg	½ tbsp cornstarch
¼ cup honey	A pinch of sea salt
½ cup milk	

DIRECTIONS and Cooking Time: 20 Minutes
Pour 1 cup of water in your IP and add a trivet. Lay pumpkin on top of the trivet. Seal the lid, and cook on Manual for 5 minutes at High. Whisk all remaining ingredients in a bowl. Do a quick pressure. Drain the pumpkin and add it to milk mixture. Pour the batter into a greased baking dish. Place in the cooker, and seal the lid. Cook for 10 minutes Manual at High. Do a quick release. Transfer pie to a wire rack to cool.

Scrumptious Stuffed Pears

INGREDIENTS for Servings: 6

3 ½ lb pears, cored	½ tsp ground cinnamon
¼ cup sugar	1 ¼ cups red wine
¼ cup walnuts, chopped	¼ cup graham cracker crumbs
¼ tsp cardamom	½ cup dried apricots, chopped
½ tsp grated nutmeg	

DIRECTIONS and Cooking Time: 20 Minutes
Lay the pears at the bottom of your cooker, and pour in the red wine. In a bowl, mix the other ingredients, except for the crackers, and pour over pears. Seal the lid, and cook Manual at High for 15 minutes. Once ready, do a quick pressure release. Top with graham cracker crumbs and serve.

White Chocolate Cake In A Cup

INGREDIENTS for Servings: 2

5 tbsp flour	4 tbsp white chocolate chips
3 tbsp sugar	4 tbsp milk
2 tbsp vanilla	3 tbsp vegetable oil
1 tsp ginger powder	
2 tbsp cocoa powder	

DIRECTIONS and Cooking Time: 15 Minutes
Pour 1 cup of water in your IP and insert a trivet. In a bowl, combine the flour, sugar, vanilla, ginger powder, milk, oil, and cocoa powder and mix well. Stir in chocolate chips. Divide the mixture between two mugs and place on the trivet. Seal the lid, press Manual, and cook for 10 minutes at High. When ready, do a quick pressure release. Serve cooled.

Grandma's Pear And Peach Compote

INGREDIENTS for Servings: 4

2 ½ cups peaches, chopped	Juice of 1 orange
	2 tbsp cornstarch
2 cups pears, diced	¼ tsp cinnamon

DIRECTIONS and Cooking Time: 2hours And 15 Minutes
Place the peaches, pears, ½ cup of water, and orange juice, in the IP. Stir to combine and seal the lid, select Manual, and set to 3 minutes at High. Do a quick pressure release. Press Sauté and whisk in the cornstarch and cinnamon. Cook until the compote thickens, for 5 minutes. When thickened, transfer to an airtight container and refrigerate for at least 2 hours.

Pumpkin Custard

INGREDIENTS for Servings: 6

2 egg yolks	1 pinch cinnamon powder
2 eggs	
2 cups pumpkin puree	1 pinch salt

½ tsp vanilla extract	2 tbsp brown sugar
1 pinch nutmeg	1 cup condensed milk

DIRECTIONS and Cooking Time: 40 Minutes
In a mixing bowl, combine all the ingredients. Pour the mixture in a greased baking dish. Add 1 cup of water in the IP and insert a trivet. Put dish on the trivet. Seal the lid, select Manual at High, and cook for 30 minutes. When done, do a quick pressure release. Serve the pumpkin custard chilled.

Authentic Spanish Crema Catalana

INGREDIENTS for Servings: 4

½ tsp cinnamon extract	½ tsp vanilla paste
1 ½ cups warm heavy cream	3 large-sized egg yolks
	1 cup sugar

DIRECTIONS and Cooking Time: 15 Minutes
In a bowl, mix cinnamon, heavy cream, sugar and egg yolks. Fill 4 ramekins with this mixture and wrap with foil. Pour 1 cup of water into the IP. Add a trivet and lay the ramekins on top. Seal the lid, press Manual, and cook for 10 minutes at High. Once the cooking is over, do a quick pressure release. Refrigerate Crema Catalana for at least 2 hours.

Cheese Fondue

INGREDIENTS for Servings: 6

1 cup Swiss cheese, shredded	2 tbsp cayenne pepper
1 clove garlic, minced	1/3 cup white wine
	4 oz cream cheese
	½ tbsp almond flour

DIRECTIONS and Cooking Time: 15 Minutes
In a glass pan, mix Swiss cheese and flour. Add in cream cheese and combine well. Stir in wine and garlic. Cover with aluminium foil. Pour 1 cup of water in the IP and put a trivet. Place the pan on top of trivet. Seal the lid and press Manual. Cook for 5 minutes at High. After cooking, do a quick pressure release. Season with cayenne pepper. When the fondue begins to thicken, merely add more wine and stir. Serve.

Hot Chicken Dip

INGREDIENTS for Servings: 4

2 chicken breasts, cubed	2 tbsp olive oil
5 oz hot sauce	1 cup ranch dressing
	16 oz cream cheese

DIRECTIONS and Cooking Time: 20 Minutes
Put the chicken, hot sauce, and ½ cup of water in the IP. Drizzle with the olive oil. Seal the lid and press Manual. Cook at High for 15 minutes. After cooking, do a quick pressure release. Remove and blend the chicken with hand mixer. Mix in the ranch dressing and cream cheese until creamy. Serve.

Zucchini Potato Patties

INGREDIENTS for Servings: 4

¼ cup coconut flakes	1 carrot, chopped
¼ cup coconut flour	½ tsp ground cumin
½ cup potatoes, mashed	1 tbsp fresh parsley
1 large zucchini, shredded	Salt and black pepper to taste
	2 tbsp olive oil

DIRECTIONS and Cooking Time: 20 Minutes
Heat oil on Sauté. Place all the remaining ingredients in a bowl. Mix with your hands until fully incorporated and then shape the mixture into 4 equal patties. Add the patties to the pot and cook for 3 minutes per side.

Coconut Stuffed Apples

INGREDIENTS for Servings: 4

2 tbsp cinnamon	½ cup coconut cream
1 cup nut butter	4 apples, cored
4 tbsp shredded coconut	A pinch of salt
	A pinch of nutmeg

DIRECTIONS and Cooking Time: 29 Minutes
Mix all ingredients, except for the apples in a bowl. Stuff the apples with this mixture. Add stuffed apples into your IP. Add 1 cup of water to the pot. Seal the lid, select Manual at High, and cook for 6 minutes. When done, release the pressure naturally for 5 minutes.

Sticky Bbq Chicken Drumsticks

INGREDIENTS for Servings: 6

3 lb chicken drumsticks	¼ cup maple syrup
2 tsp garlic, minced	2 tbsp chili sauce
¼ tsp black pepper	1 ¼ cups barbecue sauce

DIRECTIONS and Cooking Time: 30 Minutes
Arrange the drumsticks on the bottom of the IP. Add chili sauce, barbecue sauce, maple syrup, garlic, and pepper in a bowl; mix well. Pour the mixture over drumsticks in the IP. Add in ½ cup of water. Seal the lid and press Manual. Cook at High for 20 minutes. After cooking, do a quick pressure release. Serve as an appetizer.

Cinnamon & Raisin Muffins

INGREDIENTS for Servings: 4

2 eggs	¼ cup raisins
½ cup butter, softened	A pinch salt
1 cup sugar	1 cup water
¼ tsp salt	For the streusel topping:
½ tsp cinnamon	
½ tsp baking powder	¾ cup all-purpose flour
1 tsp vanilla extract	
¼ tsp nutmeg powder	½ tsp cinnamon powder

2 cups all-purpose flour	4 tbsp sugar
	¼ cup butter softened

DIRECTIONS and Cooking Time: 45 Minutes
In a bowl, beat eggs, butter, and sugar. Mix in salt, cinnamon, baking powder, vanilla extract, nutmeg, flour, and raisins. In another bowl, combine the topping ingredients. Divide the cake batter into 8 to 12 silicon muffin cups and sprinkle with the topping. Open the pot, pour in the water, insert a trivet, and place the muffin cups on top. Seal the lid and select Manual and cook for 20 minutes at High. Once done, do a natural pressure release. Let cool and serve.

Apple Cacao Dessert

INGREDIENTS for Servings: 2

1 tbsp cinnamon	1 tbsp cacao powder
1 cup apples, chopped	1 tbsp lemon juice
½ cup milk	

DIRECTIONS and Cooking Time: 13 Minutes
Place apples, cinnamon, lemon juice, and ½ cup of water in your IP. Seal the lid, select Manual at High, and cook for 3 minutes. When done, do a quick pressure release. Mix in cacao powder, and blend well.

Cremini Mushrooms With Sesame Paste

INGREDIENTS for Servings: 8

2 lb cremini mushrooms, sliced	2 tsp garlic, minced
	1 tsp cumin
2 tbsp sesame paste	2 tbsp olive oil
3 tbsp sesame seeds	Salt and black pepper to taste
1 tbsp lemon juice	

DIRECTIONS and Cooking Time: 15 Minutes
Heat oil on Sauté. Add garlic and mushrooms and cook for a minute. Pour in 1 cup of water and seal the lid. Cook on Manual for 4 minutes at High. Do a quick pressure release. Drain the mushrooms and garlic. Transfer to a food processor. Add the lemon juice, cumin, olive oil, salt, pepper, and sesame paste. Process until smooth, and stir in the sesame seeds. Serve.

Chicken Noodle Dip

INGREDIENTS for Servings: 4

2 jalapeno peppers, diced	2 cups chicken broth
	16 oz cream cheese
10 oz green chilies, diced	1 cup cooked chicken, chopped

DIRECTIONS and Cooking Time: 10 Minutes
Place all the ingredients in the IP, except for the cream cheese, then stir to combine. Seal the lid and press Manual. Cook for 5 minutes at High. After cooking, do a quick pressure release. Blend with an immersion blender. Stir in the cream cheese. Serve.

Homemade Raspberry Compote

INGREDIENTS for Servings: 4

2 cups frozen raspberries	¾ cups coconut sugar
	Juice of ½ lemon
2 tbsp arrowroot	½ cup water + 2 tbsp

DIRECTIONS and Cooking Time: 15 Minutes
Place raspberries, lemon juice, ½ cup of water, and coconut sugar in your IP. Seal the lid, cook on Manual for 3 minutes at High. Once done, do a quick pressure. Combine the arrowroot and 2 tbsp water in a bowl. Stir the mixture into the raspberries and cook until the mixture thickens, lid off on Sauté. Transfer the compote to a bowl and let chill completely before Servings .

Simple Poached Apricots

INGREDIENTS for Servings: 4

½ cup black currants	1 cup orange juice
4 apricots, pits removed	1 cinnamon stick

DIRECTIONS and Cooking Time: 10 Minutes
Place black currants and orange juice in a blender. Blend until smooth. Pour the mixture in your pressure cooker, and add the cinnamon stick. Add the apricots to the steamer basket and then insert the basket into the pot. Seal the lid, select Manual, and set to 5 minutes at High. Do a quick pressure release. Serve drizzled with sauce.

Orange Dip

INGREDIENTS for Servings: 12

1 ½ cups tofu	Salt and black pepper to taste
2 cups bok choy, chopped	
	1 ¼ cups mayonnaise
1 tsp dried dill weed	1 tsp orange zest for garnish
2 tsp fresh orange juice	

DIRECTIONS and Cooking Time: 15 Minutes
In a baking dish, mix all ingredients, except orange zest, and stir to combine. Cover the dish with aluminium foil. Pour 1 cup of water in your IP and insert a trivet. Lower the dish on the trivet. Seal the lid, and cook for 10 minutes on Manual at High. When it goes off, quick release the pressure. Sprinkle with orange zest and serve.

Crispy Potato Sticks

INGREDIENTS for Servings: 4

4 sweet potatoes, cut into sticks	3 tbsp olive oil
	1 tbsp coconut, shred
	2 tbsp almond flour

| Salt and black pepper to taste | |

DIRECTIONS and Cooking Time: 17 Minutes
Mix coconut and almond flour in a mixing bowl. Add in salt and pepper. Drizzle potato sticks with olive oil and add the coconut mixture. Stir gently. Fry the potatoes for 6-7 minutes on all sides, on Sauté. Serve.

Ice Cream Topped Brownie Cake

INGREDIENTS for Servings: 6

3 large eggs, lightly beaten	1 ½ cups sugar
1 ½ sticks butter, melted	½ cup semisweet chocolate chips
2/3 cup cocoa powder	Dash kosher salt
1 tsp pure vanilla extract	Vanilla ice cream for Servings

DIRECTIONS and Cooking Time: 60 Minutes
Line the inside of 7-inch baking dish with a piece of foil. Cover the foil with butter. In a bowl, whisk the remaining butter, flour, cocoa powder, eggs, salt, vanilla, and sugar. Fold in the chocolate chips. Pour the batter in the baking dish. Add 1 cup of water in the IP and insert a trivet. Put the dish on the trivet. Seal the lid, select Manual at High, and cook for 30 minutes. When done, perform natural pressure release for 10 minutes, then a quick pressure release to let out the remaining steam. Serve cake topped with ice cream.

Cannellini Bean & Chili Dip

INGREDIENTS for Servings: 6

4 oz cream cheese	2 oz diced green chilies
1 shallot, minced	1 cup Cannellini beans, soaked
½ tsp red pepper sauce	¼ cup Parmesan, grated
1 tsp crushed red pepper	½ cup olive oil
1 clove garlic, minced	

DIRECTIONS and Cooking Time: 40 Minutes
Put the beans and 3 cups of water in your IP. Seal the lid and press Manual. Cook for 30 minutes at High. After cooking, do a quick pressure release. Drain and place in a bowl. Add in the remaining ingredients, except for the Parmesan cheese and mix to combine. Serve topped with Parmesan cheese.

APPENDIX : RECIPES INDEX

"eat-me" Ham And Pea Soup 26

A

Alfredo Tuscan Shrimp 100
Allspice Turkey Drumsticks With Beer 70
Allspices Cake 103
Almond Butter Bars 108
Almond Butter Lemon Pears 106
Amazing White Chocolate Fondue 108
American Clam Chowder 89
Apple Cacao Dessert 113
Apple Coconut Dessert 106
Apple Coffee Cake 109
Apricot, Pear And Cherry Compote 108
Arabic-style Cauliflower Salad 48
Asian Garlic And Honey Chicken 78
Asian Vegetable Soup 15
Asian-style Chicken 80
Asian-style Flank Steaks 68
Asparagus And Mushrooms 45
Authentic French Onion Soup 28
Authentic Kentucky Burgoo 27
Authentic Spanish Crema Catalana 112
Autumn Beef Stew 60
Autumn Pumpkin Soup 30
Avocado Quinoa Salad 18
Awesome Chicken In Tikka Masala Sauce 82
Awesome Chocolate Lava Cake 106
Awesome Rutabaga And Pear Pork Loins 57

B

Bacon And Cheese Crustless Quiche 14
Bacon And Cheese Quiche 71
Bacon And Veggie Soup 32
Bacon Asparagus Wraps 111
Basil Infused Avocado Dip 103
Basil Salmon With Artichokes & Potatoes 90
Bean And Ham Soup 31
Beef & Tomato Curry 67
Beef And Cabbage Soup 37
Beef And Sauerkraut Dinner 61
Beef Borscht Soup 35
Beef Paprikash 61
Beef Ribs Texas Bbq Style 104
Beef Roast With Onions 65
Beer-steamed Mussels 96
Beets And Cheese 44
Bell Pepper & Carrot Chicken Stew 71
Bengali Parsnip Soup 24
Berry Mix, Mango And Apple Sauce 103
Best Bacon Wrapped Mini Smokies 107
Black Bean And Egg Casserole 18
Black Bean Soup 28

Borscht Beet Soup 31
Braised Collard Greens With Bacon 13
Breakfast Cobbler 22
Broccoli Leeks Green Soup 45
Broccoli With Italian-style Mayonnaise 9
Broccoli, Cauliflower & Zucchini Cakes 52
Brussel Sprouts With Onions & Apples 13
Brussels Sprout Shrimp 90
Burrito Beef 55
Buttered Chicken With Artichokes & Rosemary 78
Butternut Squash & Apple Soup 37
Butternut Squash Beef With Bok Choy 57
Butternut Squash Curry Soup 35
Buttery Mackerel With Peppers 95
Buttery Mashed Cauliflower 43

C

Cá Kho Tộ (caramelized & Braised Fish) 88
Cabbage With Carrot 50
Canned Tuna Casserole 93
Cannellini & Sausage Stew 75
Cannellini Bean & Chili Dip 114
Carrot & Chickpea Boil With Cherry Tomatoes 49
Carrot Vegan Gazpacho 48
Cashew & Tomato Soup 26
Cashew Cholocate Spread 108
Cauliflower & Potato Curry With Cilantro 51
Cauliflower Popcorn 104
Cauliflower Salad With Mozzarella Cheese 44
Celery & Red Bean Stew 51
Cheddar Baked Eggs 17
Cheddar Cheese And Broccoli Soup 36
Cheese Beef Taco Pie 64
Cheese Fondue 112
Cheese Sweet Corn 109
Cheesy Breakfast Potatoes 103
Cheesy Cauliflower Soup 26
Cheesy Chicken Quinoa 79
Cheesy Chicken Tenders 71
Cheesy Grits With Crispy Pancetta 21
Cheesy Hamburger Dip 107
Cheesy Omelet Cups 7
Cheesy Potatoes With Herbs 40
Cheesy Tomato Soup 25
Cheesy Tuna 88
Chicken & Mushrooms With White Wine 76
Chicken & Noodle Soup 36
Chicken & Vegetable Rice Soup 15
Chicken And Kale Soup 23
Chicken Congee 76

Chicken Curry (ver. 1) 70
Chicken Drumsticks With Potatoes & Veggies 75
Chicken Fricassee 70
Chicken In Garlic-mustard Sauce 84
Chicken Marrakesh 84
Chicken Noodle Dip 113
Chicken Noodle Soup 25
Chicken Salsa 85
Chicken Sandwiches With Bbq Sauce 9
Chicken Siciliano With Marsala Wine 82
Chicken Soup With Vegetables 34
Chicken Spinach Corn Soup 28
Chicken With Artichokes And Bacon 78
Chicken With Black Beans 71
Chicken With Cheese Parsley Dip 85
Chicken With Port Wine Sauce 75
Chicken, Shrimp And Sausage Gumbo 34
Chickpea & Olives Seafood Pot 87
Chickpea & Spinach Chili 27
Chickpea Hummus 19
Chili Beef Brisket With Chives 59
Chili Deviled Eggs 11
Chili-lime Shrimps 94
Chinese-style Chicken Stew With Broccoli 37
Chocolate Pudding Cake 109
Chocolate-strawberry Bars 110
Chorizo With Bell Peppers & Onions 66
Christmas Banana Bread 107
Cilantro Vegetable Beef Soup 62
Cinnamon & Raisin Muffins 112
Cinnamon-flavored Apple Sauce 103
Citrus Marinated Smelt With Okra & Cherry Tomatoes 95
Clam & Prawn Paella 92
Classic Lemon Chicken 81
Classic Mushroom Stroganoff 8
Coco Quinoa Bowl 15
Coconut & Orange Cheesecake 104
Coconut Cod Curry 88
Coconut Porridge 19
Coconut Seafood Soup 33
Coconut Stuffed Apples 112
Cod Meal 88
Codfish And Tomato Casserole 94
Collard Greens Octopus & Shrimp 95
Corn And Potato Chowder 38
Country Beef Stew With Sweet Potatoes 66
Country Chicken With Vegetables 77
Cranberry Turkey With Hazelnuts 78
Cream Of Potato Soup 7
Creamed Taco Chicken Salad 74
Creamy Artichoke, Garlic, And Zucchini 46
Creamy Chicken With Tomato Sauce 73
Creamy Mushroom Soup With Chicken 30
Creamy Spinach Tagliatelle With Mushrooms 46
Cremini Mushrooms With Sesame Paste 113
Creole Chicken With Rice 86
Crispy Potato Sticks 113
Crushed Potatoes With Aioli 53
Cuban Style Pork 63
Cumin Shredded Chicken 75
Curried Pork Stew With Peas 62

D

Delicious Chicken & Potato Soup 17
Delicious Cod With Cherry Tomatoes 90
Delicious Mushroom Goulash 48
Delicious Shrimp Salad 99
Dijon Deviled Eggs 107
Dinner Ribs With Beets And Potatoes 58
Drumsticks In Adobo Sauce 72
Duck Legs With Serrano Pepper Sauce 103

E

Easy Homemade Omelet 19
Easy Homemade Pizza 46
Easy Italian Chicken Stew With Potatoes 86
Easy Mahi Mahi With Enchilada Sauce 96
Easy Millet And Chicken Bowl 79
Easy Peach Cobbler 103
Easy Spicy Chicken Wings 79
Easy Teriyaki Chicken 76
Easy Vegan Pizza 47
Easy Vegan Posole 40
Easy Vegetarian Ratatouille 36
Easy Veggie Soup 32
Effortless Tomato-lentil Soup 14
Egg & Ham Traybake 43
Egg And Potato Mayo Salad 81
Egg Caprese Breakfast 13
Egg Noodles & Cheese With Tuna & Peas 96
Eggplant With Steamed Eggs And Tomatoes 11
Eggs & Red Beans Casserole 7
Eggs En Cocotte 7
Eggs Mushroom Casserole 12
Elegant Farro With Greens & Pine Nuts 42
English Vegetable Potage 49
Ethiopian Spinach And Lentil Soup 29
European Stew 56
Extraordinary Greek-style Fish 91

F

Fabulous Orange Chicken Stew 78
Fall Bean Chili 24
Fall Pork Loin Chops With Red Cabbage 67
Fall Root Vegetable Mix 109
Fast Chicken Rice Soup 30
Feta & Nut Green Beans 44
Fettuccine With Duck Ragout 70
Fish Packs 89
Flavorful Vegetable Mix 42
Flounder With Dill And Capers 97
French Baked Eggs 17
French Balsamic Peppers 11
Fresh Red Beets 20

Fried Turkey Meatballs With Pasta 81
Frittata With Vegetables & Cheese 16

G

Garam Masala Eggs 21
Garam Masala Parsnip & Red Onion Soup 15
Garden Vegetable Soup 17
Garlic & Leek Cannellini Beans 53
Garlic Chicken 85
Garlic Eggs 12
Garlicky Bbq Pork Butt 69
Gingered Squash Soup 25
Gingery Butternut Squash Soup 28
Glazed Baby Carrots 21
Goat Cheese & Beef Egg Scramble 16
Goat Cheese & Beef Steak Salad 22
Golden Beets With Green Olives 7
Gourmet Cilantro Salmon 17
Grandma's Noodle Soup 27
Grandma's Pear And Peach Compote 111
Grapefruit Potatoes With Walnuts 10
Greek Kakavia Fish Soup 97
Greek-style Cooked Pulled Pork 57
Green Bean Soup 30
Green Beans Salad 18
Green Chili Chicken 84
Green Chili Pork With Pomodoro Sauce 55
Green Lemon Salmon 102
Green Soup With Navy & Pinto Beans 14
Ground Pork Soup With Leeks & Carrots 57

H

Haddock Fillets With Steamed Green Beans 92
Halibut With Cheese-mayo Sauce 91
Ham And Potato Soup 29
Hard-boiled Eggs 75
Hearty Beef Soup 32
Hearty French Ratatouille 53
Hearty Irish Burgoo 35
Herbed Carp Risotto 98
Herbed Veggie Beef Rib Eye 64
Herby Cipollini Onions 105
Herby Trout Fillets With Olives 87
Holiday Almond Cake 105
Homemade Raspberry Compote 113
Homemade Turkey Burgers 73
Honey-mustard Glazed Cipollini Onions 20
Hot Chicken Dip 112
Hungarian Bean Soup 65

I

Ice Cream Topped Brownie Cake 114
Indian Coconut Kale Curry 42
Indian Dhal With Veggies 42
Indian Lentils Dhal 44
Indian Meen Kulambu 87
Electric Pressure Cooker Basic Steamed Vegetables 50
Electric Pressure Cooker Boiled Octopus 99
Electric Pressure Cooker Bread Pudding 18
Electric Pressure Cooker Cauliflower Curry 48
Electric Pressure Cooker Chicken Creole 79
Electric Pressure Cooker French Onion Soup 41
Electric Pressure Cooker Ham And Potato Soup 33
Electric Pressure Cooker Huevos Rancheros 9
Electric Pressure Cooker Lobster Roll 94
Electric Pressure Cooker Mediterranean Fish 91
Electric Pressure Cooker Steamed Artichoke 48
Instant Sweet Potato 21
Italian Stuffed Peppers With Mushroom And Sausage 14

J

Jalapeño Chicken Soup With Tortilla Chips 23
Jalapeño Ground Pork Stew 56
Japanese-style Tofu Soup 35
Juicy Chorizo Sausage With Tater Tots 64
Juicy Turkey With Mushrooms 77
Juniper Beef Ragu 68

K

Kale And Sweet Potatoes With Tofu 53
Kale And Veal Stew 32
Kale, Potato & Beef Stew 33

L

Lamb & Mushroom Ragout 63
Lamb Cacciatore 61
Lamb Shanks In Port Wine 58
Lamb With Green Onions 59
Lazy Steel Cut Oats With Coconut Milk 13
Leek Soup With Tofu 39
Lemon & Herbs Stuffed Tench 96
Lemon White Fish 98
Lemony Berry Cream 104
Lemony Chicken With Red Currants 73
Lentil & Bell Pepper Soup 38
Lentil & Carrot Chili 48
Lentil And Carrot Soup 20
Lentil-arugula Pancake 16
Light & Fruity Yogurt 11
Lime & Ginger Eggplants 46
Lime Potatoes 20
Louisiana-style Seafood Boil 95

M

Mahi-mahi With Tomatoes 89
Maple Glazed Carrots 53
Maple-glazed Acorn Squash 41
Maple-orange Glazed Root Vegetables 19
Mayonnaise & Bacon Stuffed Eggs 108
Meat Lover's Omelet 44
Meatball Soup 38
Meat-free Lasagna With Mushrooms 18
Mediterranean Cod With Cherry Tomatoes 90
Mediterranean Cod With Olives 92
Mediterranean Tomato Beef Soup 57
Mediterranean Tomato Soup With Feta Cheese 13

Mexican-style Ropa Vieja 69
Minestrone Soup 38
Mirin Tofu Bowl 51
Mix-and-match Fish Packets 98
Mixed Vegetables Medley 41
Mom's Banana Cake 110
Mom's Carrots With Walnuts & Berries 45
Mom's Orange Chicken 74
Mom's Pork Vegetable Soup 33
Mom's Rump Roast With Potatoes 59
Momma's Chicken With Salsa Verde 77
Monday Night Rice With Red Beans 54
Morning Frittatas 12
Moroccan-style Couscous Salad 19
Mount-watering Beef Ribs With Shiitake 58
Mushroom Chicken Soup 32
Mushroom Pâté 8
Mushroom-spinach Cream Soup 17
Mussels With Wine-scallion Sauce 96
Mustardy Steamed Catfish Fillets 92

O

Old Bay Crab 87
Old Bay Fish Tacos 88
Old-fashioned Duck Soup With Millet 31
Onion & Chickpea Stew 40
Orange & Red Pepper Infused Chicken 72
Orange Dip 113
Orange Marmalade Oatmeal 9
Orange-butter Sea Bass 94

P

Palak Paneer 47
Pancetta & Cheese Rigatoni 61
Papaya Short Ribs 65
Paprika Rosemary Chicken 83
Parmesan & Veggie Mash 50
Parmesan Lentil Spread 50
Parsley Pork Chili 26
Parsley Squid 99
Parsnips & Cauliflower Mash 43
Party Cinnamon & Yogurt Cheesecake 107
Peanut Pear Wedges 104
Pear Pork Tenderloin 66
Pecorino Mushroom Soup 28
Peppered Chicken With Chunky Salsa 80
Peppery Ground Pork Soup 31
Perfect Mediterranean Asparagus 15
Picante Beef Stew With Barley 63
Pilaf With Zucchini & Chicken 72
Pineapple & Soda-glazed Ham 64
Pineapple Chocolate Pudding 105
Pineapple Upside Down Cake 108
Piri Piri Chicken Soup 23
Poblano Pepper & Sweet Corn Side Dish 45
Pork & Mushrooms 63
Pork Chops In Cream Of Mushrooms 67
Pork Chops With Broccoli 65
Pork Chops With Sage 60

Pork Chops With Veggies 66
Pork City Pot 68
Pork Infused With Orange Juice 64
Pork Meatballs With Sour Mushroom Sauce 65
Pork Ribs With Tomato And Carrots 60
Pork Sandwiches 67
Pork Shoulder In Bbq Sauce 62
Pork Shoulder Infused With Lime & Mint 67
Pork Shoulder Roast With Noodles 58
Pork Soup With Red Wine 64
Pork Steaks With Apricot Sauce 66
Pork With Prune Sauce 60
Potato And Corn Soup 37
Potato Spinach Corn Mix 50
Power Green Minestrone Stew With Lemon 47
Pumpkin & Pearl Barley Soup 24
Pumpkin & Potato Mash 42
Pumpkin & Wild Rice Cajun Chicken 76
Pumpkin Custard 111
Pumpkin Hummus 109
Pumpkin Puree 43
Pure Basmati Rice Meal 51
Puréed Chili Carrots 52

Q

Quick Chicken Soup 24
Quick Indian Creamy Eggplant 45
Quick Mushroom-quinoa Soup 20
Quick Pork Chops With Cabbage 59
Quick Rum Egg Custard 110
Quick Swiss Chard & Chicken Stew 86
Quinoa Mushroom Salad 8

R

Ribs With Plum Sauce 68
Rice & Lentil Chicken With Parsley 84
Rice And Beef Soup 29
Rich And Easy Chicken Purloo 26
Rich Meatball Soup 73
Root Vegetable Stew 24
Rose Rice Pudding With Nuts 106
Rosemary Whole Chicken With Asparagus Sauce 80
Rustic Soup With Turkey Balls & Carrots 21

S

Sage Cauliflower Mash 49
Sage Chicken In Orange Gravy 83
Sage Chicken With Potatoes & Snow Beans 81
Sage Pork Butt With Potatoes 57
Sage Pork Ribs In Pecan Sauce 59
Salmon With Green Peas & Rice 100
Salmon With Parsley-lemon Sauce 87
Salmon With Pecan Coating 89
Salmon Zucchini Stew 97
Salsa Verde Chicken 71
Saucy Beef Short Ribs 61
Saucy Chicken Teriyaki 80
Sausage & Cream Cheese Dip 106
Sausage With Beer & Sauerkraut 69

Sautéed Spinach & Leeks With Blue Cheese 40
Savory Baby Back Ribs 56
Savory Beef Roast In Passion Fruit Gravy 56
Savory Chicken Wings With Worcestershire Sauce 74
Savory Spinach And Leek Relish 43
Scrambled Eggs With Cranberries & Mint 9
Scrumptious Stuffed Pears 111
Sea Scallops In Champagne Sauce 100
Sea Scallops With Champagne Butter Sauce 100
Seafood And Vegetable Ragout 33
Seafood Chowder With Bacon And Celery 34
Seafood Paella 98
Seafood Platter 93
Seafood Traditional Spanish Paella 101
Seafood With Halloumi Cheese And Olives 87
Sesame Chicken Teriyaki 82
Shredded Chicken With Marinara 83
Shrimp And Beans Mix 91
Shrimp Curry 99
Shrimp Scampi 99
Silky Lemon Cheesecake With Blueberries 110
Simple Chicken And Kale Soup 25
Simple Chicken Thighs 70
Simple Clam Chowder 23
Simple Cranberry Chocolate Biscuits 105
Simple Poached Apricots 113
Simple Steamed Salmon Fillets 90
Sliced Beef Steak With Carrots 58
Smoked Paprika Potato Chips 109
Smoky Paprika Chicken 82
Sole With Tartar Sauce 101
Soy Sauce Cheese Shrimp Scampi 100
Spanish Omelet 20
Spanish-style "tortilla De Patatas" 52
Spiced Beef Brisket & Pancetta Stew 60
Spiced Sweet Potato Soup 23
Spicy Broccoli And Cheese Soup 25
Spicy Haddock Curry 94
Spicy Honey Chicken 77
Spicy Pickled Potatoes 41
Spicy Thai Prawns 95
Spicy Vegetable Salsa 43
Spinach & Mushroom Tagliatelle 51
Spinach & Trout With Red Sauce 102
Spinach Dip 104
Spinach Hash 14
Spinach, Rice And Beef Sausage Stew 56
Spring Onion Buffalo Wings 73
Squash Tart Oatmeal 12
Steamed Artichoke 11
Steamed Artichoke With Garlic Mayo Sauce 49
Steamed Artichokes & Green Beans With Mayo Dip 45
Steamed Artichokes With Mayo Dip 46
Steamed Fish Patra Ni Maachi 99
Steamed Halibut Packets 93

Steamed Mussels In Scallion Sauce 89
Steamed Paprika Broccoli 51
Steamed Scotch Eggs 7
Steamed Trout With Garlic & Fresh Herbs 100
Steamed Vegetables 40
Steamed Vegetables Side Dish 49
Sticky Bbq Chicken Drumsticks 112
Sticky Sesame Chicken 83
Sticky Sweet Chicken Wings 111
Strawberry Compote 21
Sumac Red Potatoes 42
Sunday Beef Roast With Garam Masala 62
Sweet & Sour Pork 63
Sweet Potato Medallions With Garlic & Rosemary 52
Sweet Saucy Chicken 70
Sweet Shredded Pork 59
Swiss Chard Crisps With Orange Juice 105

T

Tagliatelle With Beef Sausage & Beans 55
Tarragon Whole Chicken 76
Tasty Apple Risotto 106
Tasty Asparagus Soup 10
Tasty Beef With Carrot-onion Gravy 61
Tasty Honey Pumpkin Pie 111
Tasty Indian Chicken Curry 84
Tasty Onion Frittata With Bell Pepper 10
Tender Bbq Ribs 59
Tender Chicken With Garden Vegetables 74
Teriyaki Chicken In Lettuce Wrap 106
Thai Coconut Curry Stew 26
Thai Tom Saap Pork Ribs Soup 31
Thanksgiving Turkey Breasts 81
The Ultimate Crab Patties 97
Three Beans Mix Chili 35
Thyme Braised Lamb Shanks 67
Thyme Creamy Beef Roast 55
Thyme Tomato Sauce 105
Tiger Prawns Paella 101
Tofu And Miso Soup 29
Tomato & Apple Cider Infused Ratatouille 47
Tomato, Lentil & Quinoa Stew 42
Traditional Locrio De Pollo 77
Traditional Provençal Ratatouille 8
Tuna With Egg 96
Tuna With Lemon And Eschalot 98
Tunisian-style Couscous 93
Turkey & Vegetable Stew 28
Turkey Fillets With Cremini Mushrooms 85
Turkey Stew With Root Vegetables 72
Turkey With Garlic Herb Sauce 85
Turkey With Smoked Paprika 80
Two-cheese Carrot Sauce 31

V

Veal And Buckwheat Groat Stew 27
Vegan Baked Beans 10
Vegan Pottage Stew 30

Vegetable Frittata With Cheddar & Ricotta 10
Vegetable Mediterranean Delight Stew 36
Vegetable Medley With Brazil Nuts 52
Vegetable One-pot 40
Vegetable Salmon Skewers 101
Vegetables With Halloumi Cheese 12
Vegetarian Chipotle Stew 47
Vegetarian Khoreshe Karafs (persian Celery Stew) 53
Vegetarian Minestrone With Navy Beans 38
Veggie Beef Steak With Beer Sauce 62
Veggie Cheese Soup 36
Veggie Flax Patties 49
Vermouth Tilapia Medley 97
Vietnamese-style Caramel Fish 93

W

Warm Spinach Salad With Eggs & Nuts 10
Well-made Cheesy Meatballs 66
White Chocolate Cake In A Cup 111
White Wine Oysters 92
Whole Chicken With White Wine 83
Winter Beef With Vegetables 68
Winter Vegetable And Lentil Stew 16

Y

Yummy Smoked Sausages 107

Z

Zesty Carrots With Pistachios 110
Zucchini & Potato Beef Stew 55
Zucchini And Bell Pepper Stir Fry 41
Zucchini Potato Patties 112

Printed in the USA
CPSIA information can be obtained
at www.ICGtesting.com
LVHW080741020824
787109LV00003B/298